Men's Health

Peter H.C. Lim
Editor

Men's Health

Springer

Editor
Peter H.C. Lim, MBBS, M Med (Surg),
M. Inst. Urol (Lon) FAMS,
D. Urol (Lon), FICS
Gleneagles Medical Centre
Singapore

Department of Urology
Changi General Hospital
Singapore

Edith Cowan University
Australia

H.T. Naval Medical School
Indonesia

ISBN 978-1-4471-4765-7 ISBN 978-1-4471-4766-4 (eBook)
DOI 10.1007/978-1-4471-4766-4
Springer London Heidelberg New York Dordrecht

Library of Congress Control Number: 2012956529

Printed on acid-free paper

Springer is part of Springer Science+Business Media (www.springer.com)

Foreword

Hypogonadism: The associations most physicians have with testosterone are that this hormone only subserves reproductive and sexual functions. Even more salient is the wrongful association most physicians assume to exist between testosterone and the development of prostate pathology such as prostate cancer and benign prostate hyperplasia. Recent studies prove otherwise and conclude that the conceptualization of the role of testosterone is based on "guilt by association," not on scientific facts. On the basis of these trepidations many more specifically amongst the elderly who is hypogonadal do not receive adequate androgen treatment.

Over the last three decades it has become apparent that the functions of testosterone in adult life are much wider than hitherto assumed. Testosterone plays a significant role in the development and maintenance of bone and muscle mass, on erythropoiesis, and on mental functions. The latter is not limited to libido but testosterone has a general vitalizing function on mood and energy. More recent are the insights that testosterone is a key player in glucose homeostasis and lipid metabolism. Again, most physicians will associate testosterone with the sex difference in cardiovascular morbidity. Cardiovascular disease and death occur about a decade earlier in the lives of men than of women. This issue has been critically reviewed and, while the sex difference undeniably exists, it cannot be attributed to testosterone *per se*. It may even be that that it is the decline of testosterone with aging that accounts for the skewed sex ratio of cardiovascular disease and death. Several studies now show that low testosterone levels are a predictor of death in elderly men. For long-time clinical conditions befalling the aging male, such as cardiovascular disease, diabetes mellitus type 2, and sexual dysfunction, were regarded as independent clinical entities. Over the last decade their close interrelationship could be convincingly demonstrated. Declining testosterone levels in the elderly, once regarded as an academic endocrinological question, appears to be central to the above pathologies. It is now clear that erectile dysfunction is an expression of endothelial dysfunction of the cardiovascular function. One could say that erectile dysfunction is a local expression in the penile vasculature of generalized vascular pathology with a common pathological basis. The common underlying factor is endothelial dysfunction. Endothelial dysfunction which manifests itself clinically as impaired vasodilation is the hallmark of erectile dysfunction. The PDE-5 inhibitors exert their pharmacological action on the endothelium improving vasodilatation. Testosterone deficiency is associated with an increased incidence of cardiovascular disease and diabetes mellitus. The latter are often the sequels of the metabolic syndrome. Visceral obesity, a pivotal characteristic of the metabolic syndrome, suppresses the hypothalamic-pituitary-testis axis resulting in lowered testosterone production. Conversely, substantial androgen deficiency leads to signs and symptoms of the metabolic syndrome. It is an omission not to include testosterone measurements in the workup of the cardiovascular disease, diabetes mellitus type 2, and erectile dysfunction. These conditions hinge on testosterone deficiency. With these recent insights, testosterone should no longer be regarded as an exotic/erotic hormone but a vital hormone for men, from the "womb to the tomb."

Premature Ejaculation: Sexual arousal accompanied by penile erection is the usual precursor to ejaculation, though not every arousal nor erection leads to ejaculation. Men typically reach orgasm 5–10 min after the start of penile-vaginal intercourse. The most significant determinant is their own sexual arousal and of their sexual partner. Most men can exercise a certain degree of control over achieving orgasm and, if they wish, may delay orgasm and ejaculation somewhat, particularly after some years of sexual experience. Premature ejaculation is the term used when ejaculation occurs before the desired time, as a rule combined with a sense of having no control over its timing.

The diagnosis hinges on the history of the patient and, in the best case, supplemented by his sexual partner. There are no laboratory tests or other diagnostic tools to verify and confirm the diagnosis. However, patients often do not present with premature ejaculation as their chief complaint. Therefore, their true problem will not be diagnosed unless a sexual history is taken. Sometimes patients present premature ejaculation as erectile dysfunction, interpreting their resolution-phase loss of erection following ejaculation as a problem of erection. Premature ejaculation may be associated with signs and symptoms of anxiety, depression, or substance abuse, as well as with difficulties or changes in the patient's relationship.

The three most commonly used clinical definitions of premature ejaculation have two basic components: an inability to control or delay ejaculation and resultant distress. The American Urological Association (AUA) 2004 guideline on premature ejaculation defines it as ejaculation that occurs sooner than desired, either before or shortly after penetration, causing distress to either partner. The American Psychiatric Association's DSM-IV further categorizes premature ejaculation as either lifelong (primary), in which the patient has rarely, if ever, been able to control ejaculation, or acquired (secondary), in which the patient initially had a period of good ejaculatory control but later in life develops premature ejaculation with all or specific partners or in specific situations. Lifelong premature ejaculation is the most common form. Acquired premature ejaculation usually begins in men between the ages of 40–50 years.

None of the three definitions stipulates objectively a "normal" time to ejaculation. In research centres where the intavaginal latency time (IELT) is used it is noted that, men with premature ejaculation will almost always have an IELT less than 4 min. The diagnosis of premature ejaculation encompasses four aspects to be considered:

- The short ejaculatory latency
- The loss of a degree of voluntary control
- The presence of marked distress or interpersonal disturbance
- Symptoms not due to any other mental, behavioral, or physical disorder

Premature ejaculation is arguably the most common form of male sexual dysfunction. The prevalence of premature ejaculation is similar across countries. In the Premature Ejaculation Prevalence and Attitudes study, 23.4–25.6 % of men in Germany, Italy, and the United States had the disorder. Frequent correlation with erectile dysfunction epidemiologic studies has found a high rate of correlation between premature ejaculation and erectile dysfunction. In the GSSAB survey, 41 % of men who reported erectile dysfunction also reported premature ejaculation, and 30 % of men reporting premature ejaculation also had erectile dysfunction. Other studies indicate that about 30 % of men with premature ejaculation also have erectile problems. Although erectile dysfunction increases in prevalence with age, premature ejaculation does not.

The above prevalence rates of premature ejaculation may be higher than many physicians would expect as most physicians do not inquire about the condition and men do not frequently offer it as a medical complaint. Underreporting of premature ejaculation is attributable to several factors including embarrassment and loss of self-esteem on the side of the patient, traditional low prioritization of the condition by the medical system, a lack of physician knowledge of premature ejaculation, and effective treatment options.

Premature ejaculation can produce significant psychological distress. Men with premature ejaculation report significantly more emotional distress, loss of self-esteem, anxiety, depression, and social isolation than men without premature ejaculation. In a study on the quality-of-life impact of premature ejaculation, 50 % of men with self-diagnosed premature ejaculation were reluctant to start a new relationship and felt distress in not satisfying their partner, and 68 % believed that their eroded sexual self-confidence and self-esteem was a primary concern.

These effects frequently take a toll on the patient's relationship with his sexual partner, often leading couples to avoid intercourse and intimacy altogether. The effects can extend beyond the purely sexual aspects of the relationship: female partners of men with premature ejaculation often report that although sex may be disappointing, they are more bothered by the break in emotional intimacy after the man has his early ejaculation. Men with premature ejaculation are often anxious, hurrying the progression of intercourse and disengaging from their partners to hide their shame. The partner sees this behavior as rejection, and both partners are often angry and frustrated. Although only 40 % of these women stated that their partner's premature ejaculation was a problem for them, 65 % of them said they would be interested in counseling and/or medication to address their partner's premature ejaculation.

Physicians may not routinely ask patients about premature ejaculation, may feel uncomfortable about asking, and may lack knowledge of the condition. Since premature ejaculation has no significant physical comorbidities, physicians may consider it a "quality-of-life" disorder and thus relegate it to a lower priority. Our current medical system strains the patient-physician relationship, often not allowing for these discussions during brief and time-pressured appointments with patients.

Persons in different societies attribute different meanings to their expressions of sexuality, and there are psychosocial and cultural connotations to the phenomenon of premature or rapid ejaculation. Certain cultural contexts may view rapid ejaculation as a sign of male prowess, and female partner sexual satisfaction may be of less significance.

Sexually Transmitted Infections in Men: Clearly because men are often the "hunters" in the sexual scheme of life and often are more promiscuous than the fairer sex and sow the seeds of sexually transmitted infections throughout the community at large from time immemorial. Sexual expression usually starts when the hormones of puberty activate the somatic substrate of sexuality and does not really end until death. Human sexuality has aspects of an instinct and a insistent recurrent biological drive, but it is influenced by mental activity and by social, cultural, educational, legal, and normative characteristics of the environment in which subjects grow up and their personality develops. It is not rare that sexually transmitted diseases are acquired in a context which breaks the above codes of behavior, such as sex outside the context of a marriage, homosexual experiences, intercourse with sex workers, and so forth and so on. The palette of human sexual behavior has many more colors than the rainbow. The relevance of the above notion is that patients with sexually transmitted diseases not only face the problem of an infectious disease but also often have strong feelings of guilt and shame. The latter may be an impediment to seek proper medical treatment.

Some religious groups oppose sex outside marriage, and object to safe-sex education programs because they believe that providing such education promotes promiscuity. Virginity pledges and sexual abstinence education programs are often promoted in lieu of contraceptives and safe-sex education programs, regarded as unnecessary when followers keep their pledge. This can place some of their members, notably teenagers, at higher risk of unintended pregnancy and sexually transmitted diseases. About 60 % of teenagers who pledge virginity until marriage do engage in premarital sex and are then one-third less likely to use contraceptives and to practice safe sex than their peers who have received more conventional sex education.

Although sexuality is very prevalent in our society today, patients may still be apprehensive about discussing details of their sexual practices. Therefore, it is imperative that we take a neutral stand on the context in which the sexually transmitted disease was acquired. The attending physician should choose his/her words carefully when taking a patient's history. It is of note that the health care provider's body language and facial expressions can discourage information disclosure. Therefore, it becomes incumbent upon the physician to create an environment free from personal prejudice in order to best serve the patient. A useful strategy may be what has become known as “the parable method.” With this method the medical caregiver relates a “parable” or a story illustrating the point that the history of the patient is not unique, and that shame or guilt in the context of treating the problem might be counterproductive in achieving diagnostic and treatment goals. Examples are “two weeks ago, I had a similar patient and this person disclosed to me… . Is that also the case with you? The information the attending physician seeks thus becomes a less personal issue of the patient who finds relief in the fact that he or she is not unique and that the attending physician obviously is at ease discussing the intimate aspects of the sexual practice that gave the patient reason to seek medical consultation. An attitude free of prejudice and moral judgment is not the same as abstaining from information and education about safe sex.

This last section covers HIV/AIDS which is fast consuming the earth if you will as the scourge of the times. It is not meant to give detailed specifics on each type of STI. Rather it covers difficult aspects e.g., How to break the unpleasant news and offers tips on counseling. The thorny issue of chronic prostatitis in Men receives special attention & tips on how to deal with depression and sexual dysfunction associated with STI’s. Finally succinct guidelines on making the diagnosis are included outside of what is learnt from medical school but most importantly how to manage the partner receives the attention this aspect deserves.

It’s far more important to know what person the disease has than what disease the person has”. If this quote of Hippocrates, the father of modern medicine, was ever true, it is in the area of diagnosing, treating and preventing sexually transmitted diseases.

Emeritus Professor Louis Gooren

Preface

Hypogonadism: The subject of hypogonadism is fraught with confusing misconceptions and controversies that the average practitioner simply cannot comprehend. Even specialists find the avalanche of information mind blogging and cannot use the conclusions drawn from them with confidence in their routine clinical practice. There was therefore a crying need for a simple, didactic text that can tell clinicians the "do's and don'ts" that are needed in the real world of clinical practice. In addition, such a book must also address the "how to do it, and what to watch out for" situations. I have tried to put together the epidemiology of the condition in the local context, the science behind the condition, its clinical presentation and the need for the correct and more accurate confirmatory laboratory tests, treatment choices and the reasons behind each preparation to use in clinical practice, safety aspects of clinical use, and hopefully an addendum of useful bedsides aids for the clinician to use in the wards or clinic. Chapters dealing with its link and use in the metabolic syndrome and erectile dysfunction have been added and covers as well the detection, use, and abuse of anabolic steroids and testosterone in sports and the thorny issue of doping. Even information on the potential use of herbal products purported to help hypogonadism has been included in this text as these products are ubiquitously used in the Asia Pacific region, and the medical practitioner must therefore have a minimum working knowledge of their pharmacology and principles behind their use.

Premature ejaculation (*PE*) is one of the most common male sexual dysfunctions, which may often be undiagnosed and undertreated due to various barriers that exist in both patients and physicians. Aside from social and cultural issues, there is also inadequate knowledge regarding available effective management strategies for PE. Information currently obtainable can be confusing and often not didactic and to the point for the ordinary practitioner who basically needs a simple "how to do it" type of cookbook by his side or clinic desk. This book is aimed to provide a simple, clear, right-to-the-point, very readable text on this subject which is not generally available. It should steer the reader through the mysteries of the pathophysiology and step by step workup on how to identify the PE patient using standard history, physical exams, and use of questionnaire instruments simple to apply at the bedside. Sections on how to use behavioral techniques and selecting the appropriate pharmacotherapy to treat the patient with primary or secondary PE, frequently asked questions, etc. are included amongst other pictorial and other useful bedsides aides.

Sexually Transmitted Infections in Men: The Management of Sexually Transmitted. Infections has become more important than ever before in this day and age especially with the growing epidemic of HIV/AIDS. The identification and treatment of infected men and more importantly the prevention of spread takes greater importance today with the world now a global village. The message of prevention and the provision of diagnostic services is emphasized in this book with advice on counseling of the patient and his partner. Whom-so-ever wishes to be a men's health doctor must be prepared to manage cases of STI's. To treat he must have passion, patience, knowledge, commitment, and zeal to handle often delicate situations. He or she must learn to create the safe space for the patient needed to admit to contracting the malady and to discuss and explore options for therapy. He must understand the challenges of trying to understand the complex physical and emotional aspects of being hit with knowing one has contracted a STI curable or non-curable. The practitioner must offer support, education, and counseling for individuals and the partner. This section is intended to provide guidance in areas not generally found in books on STI's and is not intended to be a comprehensive treatise on specific disease entities. Men's health being what it encompasses must necessarily deal with this issue.

I am grateful and honored to work with extremely distinguished scientists and clinicians known to be experts in these difficult fields of medicine and would like to put on record that without their valued contributions this book would not have seen the light of day. Finally tribute must be paid to one individual who inspired me to get thoughts onto paper and into print – Louis Gooren, MD, PhD, Professor Emeritus of Endocrinology.

Singapore, Singapore Peter Huat Chye Lim

Contents

Part III Sexually Transmitted Infections

Contributors

P. Ganesan Adaikan Ph.D., D.Sc., ACS Department of Obstetrics and Gynaecology, Yong Loo Lin School of Medicine, National University Hospital, National University of Singapore, Singapore, Singapore

Elias Tak Chuen Tam, MBBS, GDFM, GD(FP) Dermatology EHA Clinic, Shaw Centre, Singapore

Calvin Fones, MBBS, MD, FRCPsych, FAMS National University of Singapore, Gleneagles Medical Centre, Gleneagles Hospital, Singapore, Singapore

Department of Psychiatry, National University Hospital, Singapore, Singapore

Louis Gooren, M.D., Ph.D. Department of Endocrinology, Free University of Amsterdam, Amsterdam, the Netherlands

H.T. Naval Medical School, Surabaya, Indonesia

Ho Siew Hong, MBBS, MMed(Surg), FRCS, FAMS Ho Urological Clinic, Gleneagles Medical Centre, Gleneagles Hospital, Singapore, Singapore

Ng Kok Kit, MBBS (Singapore), FRCS (Glas), FRCS (Edin), FAMS (Urology) Department of Urology, Changi General Hospital, Singapore, Singapore

Andropause and Men's Health Clinic, Changi General Hospital, Singapore, Singapore

Peter Huat Chye Lim, MBBS, MMed(Surg), M.Inst.Urol(Lon) FAMS, D.Urol(Lon), FICS Department of Andrology, Urology Continence Centre, Gleneagles Hospital, Singapore, Singapore

H.T. Naval Medical School, Surabaya, Indonesia

Edith Cowan University, Joondalup, WA, Australia

Society for Men's Health Singapore, Midview City, Singapore

Gleneagles Medical Centre, Singapore, Singapore

Department of Urology, Changi General Hospital, Singapore, Singapore

Chen Yuan Tud Richard, MBBS, FRCP (Edin), FAMS Division of Endocrinology, Department of Medicine, Changi General Hospital, Singapore, Singapore

Farid Saad, DVM, Ph.D. Department of Endocrinology, Gulf Medical University & Bayer Pharma Germany, Ajman, UAE

Hang Tuah Medical University, Surabaya, Indonesia

Men's Healthcare Scientific Affairs c/o Bayer Schering Pharma AG, Berlin, Germany

Yap Seng Chong, MBBS, MRCOG, MMed(O&G), FAMS, M.D. Department of Obstetrics and Gynaecology, Yong Loo Lin School of Medicine, National University Hospital, National University of Singapore, Singapore, Singapore

B. Srilatha, M.D., Ph.D. Department of Obstetrics and Gynaecology, Yong Loo Lin School of Medicine, National University Hospital, National University of Singapore, Singapore, Singapore

Adrian Wang Chee Cheng, MBBS (Singapore), MMed (Psychiatry), FAMS Department of Psychiatry, Gleneagles Hospital Singapore, Gleneagles Medical Centre, Singapore, Singapore

Department of Psychological Medicine, National University of Singapore, Singapore, Singapore

Ng Beng Yeong Department of Psychiatry, Singapore General Hospital, Singapore, Singapore

Department of Psychiatry, Duke-NUS Graduate Medical School, Yong Loo Lin School of Medicine, National University of Singapore, Singapore, Singapore

Sin Yew Wong, MBBS, MMed(Int Med), FAMS Gleneagles Medical Centre, Gleneagles Hospital, Singapore, Singapore

Part I
Hypogonadism

Chapter 1
Epidemiology: Late-Onset Hypogonadism in Singapore

Peter Huat Chye Lim

Situation in Singapore Survey on Andropause/Late-Onset Hypogonadism

Singapore's population is aging rapidly with concurrent increase in life expectancy (74 years). Increased life expectancy and aging inflict social, health, and economic problems. A nationwide, prospective, cross-sectional, validated questionnaire-based survey was conducted in 2001 to assess andropausal symptoms and their potential implications in 228 subjects (between 45 and 70 years) of Chinese (60 %), Malay (20 %), and Indian (20 %) races. In total, 39.5 % of Singaporean males were aware of the term male menopause or andropause and 35 % signified it as normal sign of aging, requiring medical treatment (12 %). Physical- or vasomotor-associated problems were found to be more predominant (32 %) than psychological (28.9 %) and sexual (12.3 %) problems. Lack of physical energy (73.7 %) and pains in bones and joints (53.1 %) were the most commonly felt physical problems, whereas memory impairment (47.4 %) and irritability (41.7 %) constituted the psychological symptoms. Absence of nocturnal erection, lack of sexual excitement, loss of interest in sex, failures in sexual act, and poor erections dominated the sexual problems in 50.9, 42.1, 41.7, 41.2, and 38.2 % of subjects, respectively. A significant proportion

P.H.C. Lim, MBBS, MMed(Surg), M.Inst.Urol(Lon)
FAMS, D.Urol(Lon), FICS
Department of Andrology, Urology Continence Centre,
Gleneagles Hospital, Singapore, Singapore

H.T. Naval Medical School, Surabaya, Indonesia

Edith Cowan University, Joondalup, WA, Australia

Society for Men's Health Singapore, Midview City, Singapore

Gleneagles Medical Centre, Singapore, Singapore

Department of Urology, Changi General Hospital, Singapore, Singapore
e-mail: profpeter.lim@gmail.com

P.H.C. Lim (ed.), *Men's Health*,
DOI 10.1007/978-1-4471-4766-4_1, © Springer-Verlag London 2013

of population (81.2 %) reported that treatment is necessary for andropause and 45.6 % preferred treatment with a general practitioner. In Singaporean aging men, *diminishing sexual function (75 %) including ED (51.5 %) and lack of physical energy (73.7 %) were the predominant andropausal symptoms* requiring treatment. Singaporeans preferred natural approaches for andropausal symptoms (84.2 %), and 39.9 % cited treatment is not necessary. Among the andropausal symptoms in Singaporean men, lowered sexual function figured the highest and most important symptom. As the proportion of aging men likely to increase in the near future, providing better quality of life has become a necessity in these populations with the potential assessment of male menopause.

Singapore Survey on Perception of Male HRT in Singaporean Males

Hormone replacement therapy (HRT) has been accepted as a regular clinical practice in the Western world. However, the prevailing scenario with respect to HRT in Asia is still largely controversial and generally not fully accepted by the public and medical practitioners. In 2001 a nationwide, prospective, cross-sectional, validated, questionnaire-based study evaluated the perception of aging males (45–70 years) in the multiracial population of Singapore for HRT. In Singapore, only 36.8 % of aging men knew about hormone replacement and its different modalities, and 63.2 % were unaware of the same. Nearly 46 % indicated that the risk of taking hormones outweighs its potential benefits, and 46.5 % believe that hormones may lead to cancer (in particular prostate cancer). Although media (TV, radio) (26.8 %) and newspapers (30.2 %) were the main source of information on HRT, 41.7 % did not bother to get any information on HRT. Interestingly, only 10.5 % of the subjects received information from medical professionals. With respect to treatment, never, previous, and current users of HRT were 98.7, 0.4, and 0.9 %, respectively. *Lack of awareness (56.3 %) and preference for herbal treatment (23.9 %) were the main reason for higher proportion of nonusers of HRT.* Thus, the medical and social taboo about HRT in Singaporean males is high, suggesting the need for orientation and education to get men to achieve a better quality of life despite aging and late-onset hypogonadism.

Incidence of Hypogonadism in Primary Care

Incidence of hypogonadism in the population of primary care practices were assessed by a health screening. A primary care clinic-based health screening ($n = 1{,}000$) was performed in Singapore. The screening assessed androgen deficiency/hypogonadism by applying the aging male symptoms (AMS) rating scale and biochemical

Demographic variable – age:

Age Group	Total	Percentage(%)
Below 45	128	12.79
45–49	127	12.69
50–54	195	19.48
55–59	212	21.18
60–64	141	14.09
65–69	77	7.69
Above 69	51	5.09
NA (age not available)	70	6.99
Mean		54.70

Fig. 1.1 Age distribution of hypogonadism patients

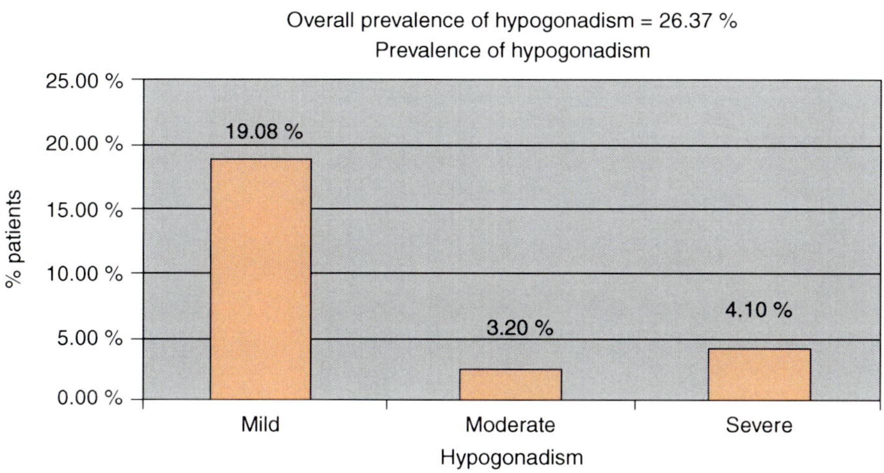

Fig. 1.2 Prevalence of hypogonadism in Singapore

quantification of testosterone level. In addition, the sexual health function was also further elucidated by the International Index of Erectile Dysfunction (IIEF) scores.

Of the 1,000 patients screened between 17 Oct 2007 and 30 Sept 2009, the mean age of the population was 54.7 years (Fig. 1.1), and nearly *26.37% were noted to have some form (mild, moderate, and severe) of androgen deficiency* according to the AMS rating scale (Fig. 1.2). Of this, 19.08 % had mild deficiency, 3.2 % had moderate deficiency, while severe deficiency was identified in 4.10 % of respondents. With respect to age, higher incidence was determined in men above 69 years of age (43.4 %, odds ratio 3.44), whereas men between the age of 45 and 69 had an average incidence of (17.9 %, odds ratio 0.91). The primary medical conditions among the survey population were diabetes, hyper-cholesterol, hypertension, obesity, and prostate problems, respectively, in 17, 33, 35, 26, and 5 %, while *androgen deficiency*

Medical conditions and odds ratio of developing hypogonadism

	YES		NO	
	Odds ratio	*p*-value	Odds ratio	*p*-value
Cigarette smoking	0.163	<0.001	6.143	<0.001
Exercise	65.000	<0.001	184.000	<0.001
Overweight	6.267	<0.001	9.333	<0.001
High cholesterol	5.368	<0.00	16.842	<0.001
Drug allergy	3.857	<0.001	31.286	<0.001
Hypertension	18.000	<0.001	23.333	<0.001
Diabetes	9.429	<0.001	25.857	<0.001
Prostate problem	0.680	0.220	8.360	<0.001
Erectile dysfunction	12.824	<0.001	0.078	<0.001

odds ratio reveal that medical factors such as smoking, exercise, overweight, high cholesterol, hypertension, diabetes and ED have higher odds of developing hypogonadism

Fig. 1.3 Medical conditions and risk of hypogonadism

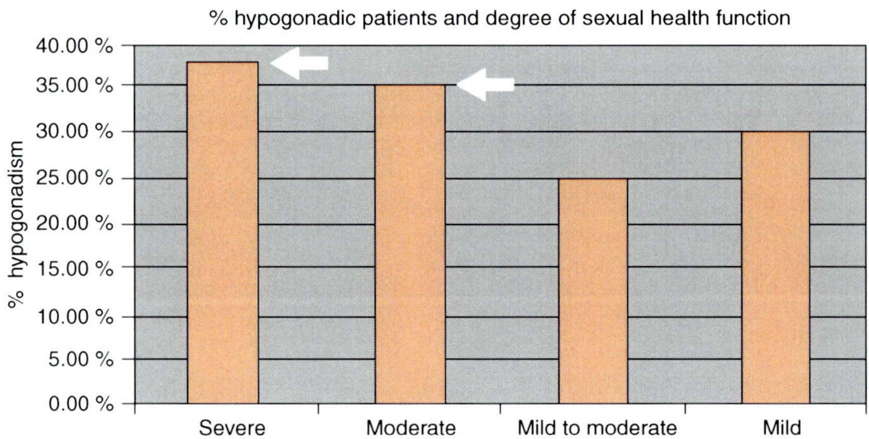

Fig. 1.4 Hypogonadism patients and degree of sexual health function

was 38, 25, 24, 28, and 30 % in people with diabetes, hyper-cholesterol, hypertension, obesity, and prostate problems, respectively (Fig. 1.3). The survey highlighted that our Singapore population had more physiological (97 %) and sexual problems (95 %) compared to psychological (91 %). Sexual function as assessed by AMS rating scale showed that only 6.3 % had a normal function and 90.2 % had below-average function. Of this, 20 and 11.4 % were androgen deficient at below-average and normal sexual function, respectively. Sexual function was further analyzed by IIEF scores and severe, moderate, mild to moderate, and mild ED were 36.1, 31.4, 22.8, and 6.3 %, respectively, and in this population the presence of androgen deficiency was 37.2, 35.1, 24.9, and 30 % at these grades of ED (Fig. 1.4).

These results highlight that diabetes and prostate disorders have greater influence on the status of androgen deficiency and its associated disorders compared to other medical conditions. Androgen deficiency impacts significantly on physiological and sexual function. Hence, a greater awareness of the condition and a crying need for remedial measures for androgen deficiency or hypogonadism is warranted as it has significant effect on overall health and well-being in Singaporean men in view of the aging population in Singapore.

Bibliography

Lim PHC. Results from a men's health screening for hypogonadism in Primary Health Care – 1000 men with clinical & biochemical diagnostic confirmation. Project of the Society for Men's Health Singapore, Singapore. 2007–2009.

Quek P, Khin LW, Lim PHC. National survey on knowledge, attitudes and practices relating to "Andropause" in Singapore. Joint project of MRC, Clinical Trials & Epidemiology Research Unit, Min of Health & the Society for Men's Health, Singapore. 2001.

Chapter 2
Pathophysiology of Late-Onset Hypogonadism and Risks and Benefits of Replacement Therapy

Peter Huat Chye Lim

Introduction

The testosterone molecule is depicted below (Fig. 2.1).

Testosterone is primarily produced by Leydig cells of the testicles in response to LH (luteinizing hormone) stimulation from the pituitary gland, and within the target cell, it is broken down into DHT (dihydrotestosterone) and E2 (estradiol). DHT is the active component which gives the androgenic effects. The adrenal glands mainly produce its precursor dehydroepiandrosterone (DHEA) and contribute a small amount of testosterone to the sum total. In utero during development the effects of testosterone on the target organs are depicted in Fig 2.2.

P.H.C. Lim, MBBS, MMed(Surg), M.Inst.Urol(Lon)
FAMS, D.Urol(Lon), FICS
Department of Andrology, Urology Continence Centre,
Gleneagles Hospital, Singapore, Singapore

H.T. Naval Medical School, Surabaya, Indonesia

Edith Cowan University, Joondalup, WA, Australia

Society for Men's Health Singapore, Midview City, Singapore

Gleneagles Medical Centre, Singapore, Singapore

Department of Urology, Changi General Hospital, Singapore, Singapore
e-mail: profpeter.lim@gmail.com

P.H.C. Lim (ed.), *Men's Health*,
DOI 10.1007/978-1-4471-4766-4_2,

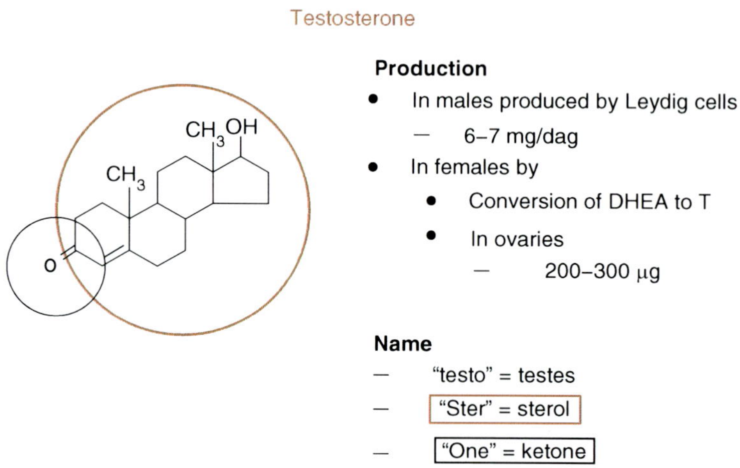

Fig. 2.1 Molecular structure of testosterone

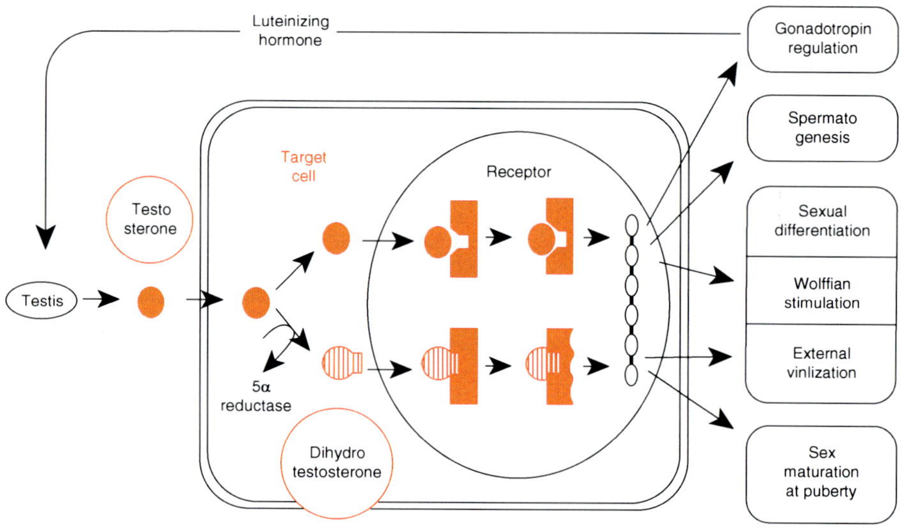

Fig. 2.2 Testosterone and its effects on various target organs (Griffin 1992)

Testosterone: Physiological Effects

- CNS – libido, energy, spatial cognition, well-being, memory
- Larynx – lowers voice
- Liver – lowers SHBG and HDL
- Kidney – raises erythropoietin

- Prostate – increases size and secretions
- Genitals – development, erections, spermatogenesis
- Skin – increases facial and body hair and sebum production
- Blood – increases hematocrit
- Adipose tissue – increases lipolysis, decreases abdominal fat
- Bone – increases bone mineral density
- Muscle mass – increases lean mass and strength

Sexual Effects

Testosterone, acting at multiple sites to maintain sexual activity, enhances sexual interest and libido in addition to its local effects on erectile function. It was previously thought that its main action targets sexual interest and libido primarily, but recent data demonstrates local effects for erectile function in respect of expression of NOS in penile tissue which is dependent on androgens. Castration affects PDE5 gene expression, and PDE5i efficacy is seen to be blunted in patients with hypogonadism. Thus, our concept of the pathophysiology of ED has changed, and today we note that testosterone deficiency produces metabolic, structural, and functional alterations in the corpus cavernosum resulting in veno-occlusive dysfunction and explains why PDE5 inhibitors are less effective in ED patients with testosterone deficiency. In animal models, androgen deficiency produces increased accumulation of adipocytes in the sub-tunical region of the corpus cavernosum causing veno-occlusive dysfunction which cannot be restored with PDE5 inhibitors treatment alone.

Mood and General Well-Being

Adequate testosterone is needed for general and mental well-being (data relating mood to serum testosterone divergent). Recent Epidemiologic data showed depressed mood inversely related to bioavailable testosterone. Testosterone replacement in aging men improved general well-being.

Androgens and CVS Diseases

Epidemiologic data showed increased CVS diseases with low serum testosterone levels. Androgen replacement produced a small but significant reduction in HDL cholesterol. Clinical significance of this is unknown. Testosterone has been shown to have direct vasodilatory effects on coronary vessels. Other lipid, coagulation, fibrinolytic, and hormonal factors are changed with use of testosterone.

Central Nervous System

Androgens can affect release of neurotransmitters and modulate neuronal nicotinic receptors. It may interact with acetylcholine binding and thus affect cognition by enhancing hippocampal acetylcholine release and modulating nicotinic acetylcholine receptors. In castrated rats, there is reduced total spontaneous release of acetylcholine.

Thus, serum testosterone correlates with cognitive function and spatial ability in men, and androgen replacement in elderly men improves spatial ability but no effect on memory or verbal fluency.

Bone Mineral Density

When testosterone is split into DHT (dihydrotestosterone) and E2 (estradiol), the E2 maintains good BMD for patients. In hypogonadic males, there is an increased risk of osteopenia and osteoporosis, leading to greater prevalence of femoral neck fractures and compression fractures of the thoracolumbar spine during falls and minor traumata.

Muscle

Testosterone maintains muscle strength and mass and prevents frailty of aging.

Etiopathogenesis of Late-Onset Hypogonadism

Several mechanisms of age-associated decrease in androgen levels have been postulated:

- Primary testicular changes
- Altered neuroendocrine regulation of Leydig cell function
- Increase of SHBG binding capacity
- Decreased adrenal androgen secretion

Primary testicular changes may cause the following:

- Decreased secretary capacity of Leydig cells
- Reduction of number Leydig cells
- Reduction of enzymes
- Shift from $\Delta 5$ to $\Delta 4$ steroids

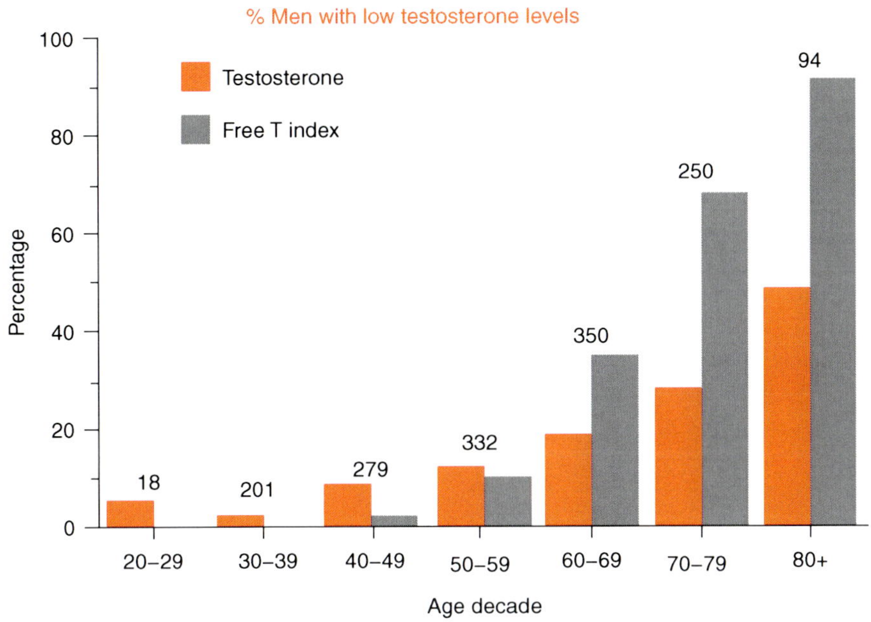

Fig. 2.3 Declining testosterone with age (Harman et al. 2001)

Altered neuroendocrine regulation of Leydig cell function leads to:

- Modestly and inconsistently higher LH levels
- Slightly increased LH response to GnRH
- Unchanged pulsatile LH secretion
- Diminished frequency of large amplitude LH pulses
- Reduced mean LH pulse amplitude
- Increased responsiveness to negative feedback of androgens
- Decreased hypothalamic GnRH secretion (Figs. 2.3 and 2.4)

Late-Onset Hypogonadism (LOH): Clinical Presentation

In late-onset hypogonadism, the male patient may experience:

- Diminished sense of well-being and energy
- Diminished libido and frequency of intercourse
- Decreased muscle mass and strength
- Increased fat mass + altered distribution
- Decreased skin thickness and male-pattern hair distribution
- Osteopenia/osteoporosis

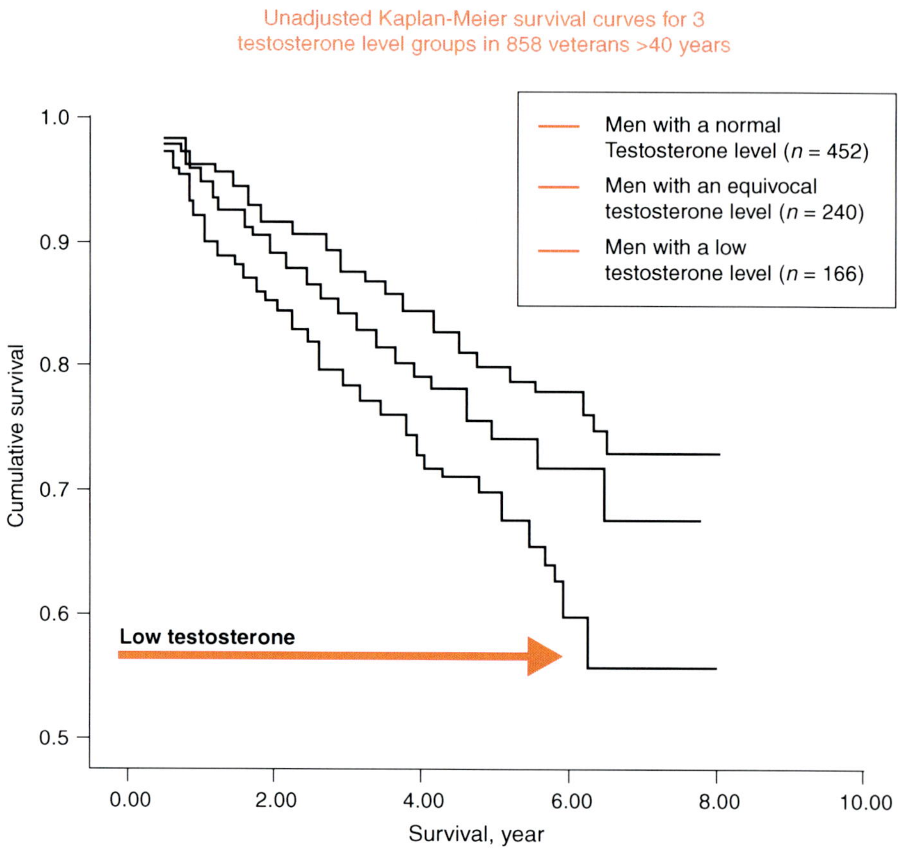

Fig. 2.4 Testosterone levels and survival (Shores et al. 2006)

Benefits of Testosterone Replacement for Men

- Sex drive/potency increase
- Cardiovascular system improvement
- Circulatory system improvement
- Muscular strength improvement
- Cholesterol profile improvement; potential reduction in risk of coronary heart disease
- Leaner body mass
- Improved self-perceived wellness
- Minimization of bone loss
- Stabilization of blood sugar
- Hematological improvement
- Prevention of peripheral vascular disease, muscle cramps, liver dysfunction, Alzheimer's disease
- Improvement of pregangrenous conditions

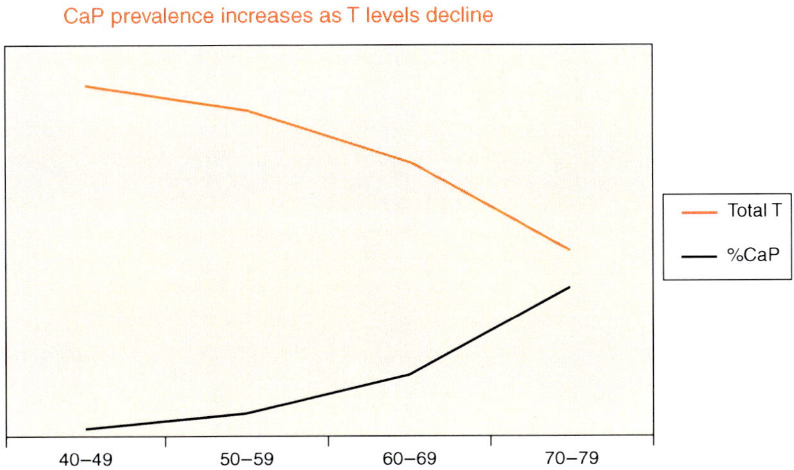

Fig. 2.5 Cancer of the prostate prevalence and testosterone levels

Potential Risks of Replacement Therapy

BPH

- Hypogonadal men have small prostates.
- In hypogonadal men receiving testosterone treatment, prostatic volume increases, but to no greater volume than that of normal age-matched controls.
- PSA levels rise with androgen therapy but should remain within the reference range.
- Maximal increase in volume and PSA occurs by 3 months and does not continue with long-term therapy.

Prostate Carcinoma

- There is no evidence that testosterone treatment causes prostate cancer.
- Testosterone seems to be a "permissive" rather than a "causal" factor.
- This issue is still controversial, but current evidence points to older men with low testosterone being at higher risk of getting carcinoma of the prostate (Fig. 2.5).

Cardiovascular Risk

- Both androgen deficiency and androgen excess are associated with unfavorable lipid profiles and increased CV risk.
- Maintaining androgen levels in the physiological range promotes a favorable lipid profile.

- Early studies have been conducted in hypogonadal men with angina and chronic heart failure showing benefit from normalization of testosterone levels.
- More research is needed on CV risk.

Polycythemia

- Clinically significant polycythemia has been associated with androgen replacement.
- This is more common with conventional injectable (up to 44 %) therapy, where high peak plasma concentrations are found immediately after administration.
- Much less common with transdermal (8 %) therapy or long-acting injection (Nebido).

Liver

- Only alkylated testosterone preparations have been associated with liver disease
- Modern testosterone preparations, either biologically identical testosterone or testosterone esters, are not associated with liver disease.

Other Side Effects

- Other less common side effects are acne, male-pattern hair loss, hirsutism, mood changes, and rarely sleep apnea.

Conclusion

- Decreasing testosterone levels are associated with a decline in:
  - Libido and sexual function
  - Bone mineral density
  - Lean body mass and muscle strength
- Replacement studies in elderly men with *mildly low* testosterone levels have not convincingly shown a benefit or reversal of these changes.
- However, in elderly men with very low testosterone levels (<200–300 ng/dl), there is improvement in libido and BMD and possible improvement in sexual function and the perception of physical well-being.

- Testosterone replacement mildly increases PSA levels and may exacerbate androgen-dependent diseases (BPH and prostate cancer if present and not picked up before starting therapy) which increase with age. However, clinical studies to date are too small to determine any clear adverse effect in the ordinary patient suitable for replacement therapy.
- Testosterone replacement can cause erythrocytosis which therefore mandates a check on the hematocrit during long-term therapy.

References

Griffin JE. Androgen resistance the clinical and molecular spectrum. N Engl J Med. 1992;326: 611–18.

Harman SM, et al. Body Composition, Metabolic Syndrome & Testosterone in Aging. J Clin Endocrinol Metab. 2001;86:724–31.

Shores MM, et al. Low Testosterone & Mortality in Male Veterans. Arch Intern Med. 2006;166: 1660–5.

Chapter 3
Testosterone Assays and Their Potential Pitfalls

Chen Yuan Tud Richard

The ideal hormonal assay would be one that is inexpensive, widely available and easy to perform, and yields stable and highly reproducible results with excellent accuracy without being susceptible to external factors.

Testosterone assays, though easily available and inexpensive, pose a number of challenges. Several considerations must be taken into account:

- Physiological state of testosterone: The majority of testosterone is bound to a carrier protein, rendering the hormone inactive. Fifty percent is tightly bound to sex hormone-binding globulin (SHBG) and about 45 % less tightly bound to albumin. Some dissociation is possible from the latter fraction, which may possess some biological activity. Only the remaining 3–4 % is unbound, also termed free testosterone (FT), which is biologically active. The frequently performed total testosterone (TT) assay measures all three fractions:

$$TT = [T{\cdot}SHBG] + [T{\cdot}Albumin] + FT$$

$$BT = [T{\cdot}Albumin] + FT$$

  It would be ideal if it is possible to measure the tiny FT fraction accurately and easily, but this is technically difficult. How much of the albumin-bound fraction is biologically active is also unclear. Some workers opt to measure this fraction *and* FT, collectively termed as bioavailable testosterone (BT). Again, accurate assays for BT are technically difficult. Overall, there is, perhaps, more experience with FT than there is for BT.

Much of the material in this chapter has been adapted from the paper by: Rosner W, Auchus RJ, Azziz R, Sluss PM, Raff H. Position statement: utility, limitations, and pitfalls in measuring testosterone: an Endocrine Society position statement. J Clin Endocrinol Metab. 2007;92(2):405–13.

C.Y.T. Richard, MBBS, FRCP (Edin), FAMS
Division of Endocrinology, Department of Medicine,
Changi General Hospital, Singapore, Singapore
e-mail: richard_chen@cgh.com.sg

P.H.C. Lim (ed.), *Men's Health*,
DOI 10.1007/978-1-4471-4766-4_3, © Springer-Verlag London 2013

- The impact of SHBG: As a large proportion of testosterone is significantly bound to SHBG, fluctuations in SHBG will directly influence the overall value of TT. Most commonly, levels of SHBG tend to be higher with increasing age and lower in obese persons. Conditions such as hyperthyroidism, cirrhosis, anticonvulsant usage, and hypogonadism itself also cause elevation in SHBG, while hypothyroidism, glucocorticoid usage, nephrotic syndrome, and androgen therapy depress SHBG levels (Tung and Cunningham 2007). As such, it is important to take into account SHBG concentrations when assessing androgen status.
- Lack of standardization: A major problem is the lack of a reference standard across different laboratories and equipment manufacturers, even for the same assay method. This hinders the exact determination of accuracy.
- Assay interference: Presence of other steroids with similar structure may cause assay interference.

Basic Technical Aspects of Common Assay Methods

1. *Radioimmunoassay* (*RIA*): A sensitive method used to assay small quantities of an antigen, typically a hormone. Firstly, an antigen (e.g., testosterone) is labeled with a radioactive isotope. This is then mixed with a known quantity of antibody specific for the antigen, with which it binds. Serum from the patient containing unknown quantities of that same antigen is added, competing with the radiolabeled antigen for binding sites on the antibody, displacing the latter. As more of the patient's serum is added, more of the radiolabeled antigen is displaced. The latter is then separated from the bound antigen, and the amount of radioactivity measured. A binding curve is generated using known standards, from which the quantity of the patient's antigen (testosterone) is derived. However, because of the usage of radioactive substances, RIA can only be conducted in facilities licensed to handle nuclear material, especially the safe disposal of radioactive waste.
2. *Chemiluminescent enzyme immunoassay* (*CLIA*): The basic methodology involves the generation of light energy from a reaction (usually involving the use of peroxidase), which is amplified and measured. The principle shares some common ground with RIA: unknown quantities of testosterone from the patient's serum compete with a testosterone-peroxidase conjugate to bind to a known quantity of anti-testosterone antibody. As more of the endogenous testosterone is added, more testosterone-peroxidase conjugate is displaced. The displaced conjugate is removed and added to a chemiluminescent substrate. A reaction takes place where light is produced, the amount emitted being proportional to the amount of peroxidase present, and inversely proportional to the amount of endogenous (patient's) testosterone, which is derived from a binding curve in the same manner as RIA above. As CLIA does not involve radioactivity and provides a high degree of accuracy, this is currently one of the most widely used methods commercially nowadays, superseding conventional colorimetric methods such as enzyme-linked immunosorbent assay (ELISA).

Total Testosterone

Measurement of total testosterone (TT) is central to almost all other methods of quantifying testosterone, as they rely on the value of TT obtained. As such, a robust technique is necessary.

Most commercial- and hospital-based laboratory assays employ the direct method by RIA or CLIA. These methods are rapid, technically simple and inexpensive to perform. However, the shortcomings are that reference ranges are not well established, and it lacks accuracy at low testosterone concentrations, below 10 nmol/L, which may be a problem when assessing androgen status in older men in the context of andropause, as there is a tendency toward overestimation.

A more accurate method would be to perform additional procedures of *extraction and chromatography*, before proceeding with RIA. By removing interfering proteins and separation of cross-reacting steroids, the final assay sample is much "cleaner", offering greater sensitivity and accuracy. However, this method is highly time-consuming and labor intensive and can only be performed in facilities licensed to carry out work involving radioactive substances.

A variation of the above is using *mass spectrometry* (*MS*), instead of RIA, after extraction and chromatography. This is, nowadays, regarded as the likely gold standard. Nevertheless, it remains expensive and time-consuming, which relegates these elaborate methods mostly for research purposes only.

Free Testosterone

Free testosterone (FT), being the active unbound fraction, correlates better with androgen status than total testosterone. It is the preferred measure of testosterone (in the same vein as free thyroxine), if it can be quantified accurately. As the fraction of FT is tiny, extremely accurate assays are needed.

A common commercial assay is direct RIA (also known as analog method), which is automated, rapid, and inexpensive. However, it lacks the sensitivity to measure the tiny fraction due to significant binding of analog to serum proteins, hence yielding poor accuracy. It is best avoided.

The gold standard is *equilibrium dialysis*, otherwise known as the indirect method. A radioactive tracer ^{3}H-testosterone is added to the assay sample, after which protein-bound testosterone, as well as other impurities, are physically separated using a membrane or via ultrafiltration, allowing the remaining tracer attached to FT to be measured. This is then multiplied by the amount of total testosterone, assayed separately from the same plasma. Although accuracy is excellent, this method is necessarily time-consuming and labor intensive, requiring a licensed nuclear facility. As such, it is mostly employed only in research settings. The accuracy of equilibrium dialysis is highly dependent upon the accuracy of TT, which is a critical variable.

Fortunately, a very convenient way of estimating FT without the need for cumbersome methodology is available – through *calculation*, using values of TT, SHBG, albumin, and the equilibrium dissociation constants of the binding of SHBG and albumin to testosterone. Nowadays, an online calculator is available (http://www.issam.ch/freetesto.htm). Calculated FT (CFT) correlates very well with actual values of FT obtained through equilibrium dialysis, making it a highly useful tool for assessing androgen status in older men.

Some older literature mentions the use of the Free Androgen Index (FAI), expressed as percent and calculated from the fixed formula:

$$(T \div SHBG) \times 100.$$

The FAI is quite appropriate in women, where the Law of Mass Action is valid, as testosterone concentrations are very low. In men, however, the much higher concentration of testosterone exceeds the binding capacity of SHBG, thus invalidating the Law of Mass Action. As such, the FAI correlates poorly with FT in men and is not recommended.

What Investigations to Order and When?

Given the considerations above, it is clear that *TT* and *SHBG* are essential measurements. The SHBG value provides some perspective to the TT level. For instance, the TT value in an older male may appear to be well within the normal range because the corresponding SHBG is elevated.

Knowing both the TT and SHBG values also allows one to calculate the free testosterone concentration, which is especially useful when assessing androgen status in older males, where TT values are often borderline low, and may be influenced by SHBG concentrations as well. If possible, the serum *albumin* value (usually part of liver function testing) should be obtained as well, as it is a component in the calculation of FT. In the same manner as SHBG, higher levels of albumin will elevate TT levels and vice versa.

It is also a good practice to obtain values of *luteinizing hormone* (*LH*) and *follicle-stimulating hormone* (*FSH*) as well, as this allows the clinician to ascertain, should the patient really have hypogonadism, whether it is due to testicular or pituitary dysfunction.

The *timing* of these investigations is absolutely critical. Testosterone is secreted in a circadian fashion. Levels are highest in the early hours of the morning, after which they decline. In fact, sampling after 10:00 a.m. will probably turn out to be unreliable. As such, early morning sampling is absolutely imperative, and at least two samples should be obtained on separate occasions to demonstrate consistency in results.

Case Study 1
An 18-year-old male, perfectly healthy, was seen by a physician because of mild gynecomastia. Apart from that, there was no other clinical sign to suggest that he may be hypogonadal, as he appeared well virilized. An androgen panel was conducted which initially showed TT 14.4 nM and FT (direct) 33.9 pM (the lab's reference range

being 40–47 pM). As the FT appeared lowish, the panel was repeated again several months later at 3:00 p.m., which showed TT 15.8, FT (direct) even lower at 25.3, SHBG 49 nM, and albumin 44 g/L. The calculated free testosterone (CFT) was 250 pM, which seemed low for such a healthy young man. By then, his gynecomastia had long subsided spontaneously. He was referred to the author, whereupon a proper assessment was performed at 9:00 a.m. This time, the results unequivocally showed this young man to be perfectly normal: TT 21.0 and CFT 426, based on a SHBG of 40.5 and albumin 41.

This case demonstrates several important points in the assessment of androgen status:

- Early morning blood samples are essential.
- Know the type and quality of the assay being used and the properly established and validated reference intervals. In this example, the direct (analog) FT is a poor assay, and the "reference range" provided was dubious. This assay should *never* be used at all.
- Diagnosis is not based on numbers alone. The biochemical result must correlate clinically. The fact that this young man did not appear hypogonadal should have alerted the clinician that the results were spurious.

Case Study 2
A 52-year-old man, previously healthy, complains of reduced libido, erectile dysfunction, reduced drive and energy, and poorer concentrating ability. An assessment showed TT 18.4 nM and SHBG 64.8 nM (ref: 15–50). This level of TT seemed very adequate, but in fact, it is misleadingly so because his SHBG is elevated. His calculated FT turned out to be only 239 pM, well below the level expected of his age. After receiving androgen therapy, his posttreatment results were the following: TT 18.3, SHBG 46.5, and CFT 326. Although his TT remained static, his SHBG has decreased with androgen therapy, resulting in a higher concentration of CFT, along with a significant improvement in symptoms.

This case illustrates how SHBG can influence TT levels and, hence, the importance and usefulness of CFT in assessing androgen status. The issue of reference ranges will be discussed in Chap. 4.

Reference

Tung DS, Cunningham GR. Androgen deficiency in men. Endocrinologist. 2007;17:101–15.

Chapter 4
Diagnosing and Evaluating Androgen Deficiency, Including Andropause

Chen Yuan Tud Richard

The diagnosis of an endocrine problem should satisfy the following: the clinical features, comprising symptoms, and signs (if present) must be consistent; biochemically, the level of the hormone concerned must be shown to be inappropriately below the age- and gender-specific reference ranges.

This principle applies equally to androgen deficiency. However, certain difficulties abound. The symptoms and signs are highly variable, and age-specific reference ranges are not well established. Furthermore, due its physiological properties, there is debate over which form of testosterone to measure, and available assay methods may not be adequately robust or not widely available.

This chapter addresses the following:

1. Classification of androgen deficiency
2. Clinical features
3. Likely reference ranges
4. Diagnostic criteria
5. The implications of androgen deficiency in older men

Classification of Androgen Deficiency

A more useful way is to adopt a functional classification, where the problem may either be true androgen deficiency or relative androgen deficiency.

C.Y.T. Richard, MBBS, FRCP (Edin), FAMS
Division of Endocrinology, Department of Medicine,
Changi General Hospital, Singapore, Singapore
e-mail: richard_chen@cgh.com.sg

P.H.C. Lim (ed.), *Men's Health*,
DOI 10.1007/978-1-4471-4766-4_4,

True Androgen Deficiency

A male subject may be labeled with true androgen deficiency when the diagnosis is beyond reproach: he exhibits some clinical features of hypogonadism that are consistent with unquestionably low levels of serum testosterone.

The etiology may either be primary or secondary hypogonadism. In the former, the pathology lies with testicular dysfunction, resulting in elevated serum concentrations of gonadotrophins luteinizing hormone (LH) and follicle-stimulating hormone (FSH) in the presence of low serum testosterone. This is also referred to as hypergonadotrophic hypogonadism.

In secondary hypogonadism (hypogonadotrophic hypogonadism), the hypothalamus or pituitary gland is at fault, resulting in gonadotrophins that are either low or inappropriately normal, in the presence of low serum testosterone.

Age-Related Relative Androgen Deficiency

Age-related relative androgen deficiency, on the other hand, refers to a proportion of middle-aged (or older) men who experience symptoms similar of androgen deficiency, and are found to have levels of serum testosterone that are low for age, in the absence of any clear pathological cause. This phenomenon has also been variously termed late-onset hypogonadism or partial androgen deficiency of the aging male (PADAM) or, the best known, andropause. These men are, otherwise, quite healthy and free of any chronic debilitating disease. At most, they may only suffer from mild hypertension or dyslipidemia, under treatment, and they are taking no more than two different classes of prescription drugs. This distinction is important, as it would exclude older men with low serum testosterone in the presence of chronic diseases such as diabetes mellitus, heart failure, and renal and hepatic failures.

It is important to differentiate andropause from men, of similar age, whose serum testosterone concentrations appear to be low for age but who are symptom-free. The clinical significance of low serum testosterone per se, without accompanying symptoms, in men who are otherwise healthy is presently unclear. There is data showing that androgen deficiency is associated with poor metabolic status and higher risk of new-onset type 2 diabetes mellitus (Stellato et al. 2000; Chen et al. 2006; Laaksonen et al. 2003). Very low serum concentrations of total testosterone have also been linked with higher mortality risk, independently of age and other cardiovascular risk factors (Laughlin et al. 2008). However as there is insufficient data showing outcomes with long term testosterone therapy, there is little justification to treat men with numerically low serum testosterone levels in the absence of symptoms or pathology related to androgen deficiency.

It is important to appreciate that true and relative androgen deficiencies represent polar ends of the clinical spectrum of androgen deficiency. If untreated, they lead to similar consequences: poorer metabolic status, central adiposity, osteopenia, reduced libido, and psychosomatic complaints, viz., reduced drive, energy, and motivation, depression, and mood swings.

Clinical Features of Androgen Deficiency

The clinical features of hypogonadism are determined by several factors: age of onset, duration, and the biochemical severity of androgen deficiency. Generally, clinical signs, if present, are more reliable indicators of androgen deficiency than symptoms, which may be quite nonspecific.

Gynecomastia, whether unilateral or bilateral, frequently accompanies significant androgen deficiency, regardless of etiology.

The classic appearance of a "young-for-age" male lacking in secondary sexual characteristics and male body hair distribution, with pale nipple areola, small testicular volume, and micropenis, is only found if hypogonadism occurred during the prepubertal years.

On the other hand, onset of hypogonadism during adolescence around the pubertal period may result in the subject being tall, due to delayed fusion of the epiphyses of the long bones. After some duration, subjects are likely to develop a eunuchoidal habitus, where arm span exceeds height, pubis-heel length exceeds pubis-crown length, body hair is sparse, and body contour around the hips is distinctly more feminine. Klinefelter syndrome is probably the most classic, and commonest, example with such clinical features.

Isolated hypogonadotrophic hypogonadism (Kallmann syndrome) may be associated with some unique features, viz., tall stature, anosmia, and midline facial defects such as cleft lip and palate.

Hypogonadism of adult onset, occurring well after puberty, is usually due to some pathological process, causing direct testicular dysfunction or affecting the hypothalamo-pituitary-gonadal axis. The clinical features are much more subtle, very much depending on the duration, and degree of severity, of biochemical hypogonadism. Signs of virilization will, of course, remain, but with time, the pubic and axillary hair may appear more sparse, and testicular volume may shrink. Gynecomastia may eventually appear.

The range of clinical symptoms may be extremely wide. Hypogonadal men may remain relatively asymptomatic. On the other hand, they may experience symptoms such as reduced energy levels, reduced libido, and lack of motivation, which have been reported as the three commonest symptoms of hypogonadal men (Laughlin et al. 2008). Other complaints include hot flushes, sleep disorders, easy fatigability, mood swings, and poorer concentrating ability.

It is important to note that hypogonadism may not necessarily be accompanied by erectile dysfunction. While testosterone stimulates endothelial nitric oxide synthase, as well as androgen receptors in parasympathetic dilator nerves, and fuels libido (sexual thoughts and fantasies), direct tactile penile stimulation per se, which is androgen independent, can also lead to an erection.

Are Symptoms of Androgen Deficiency Quantifiable?

The self-administered Aging Males' Symptoms (AMS) scale (which has been validated in different languages and cultures, including Asia, and available from http://www.issam.ch) is frequently used to quantify the severity of the symptom complex experienced by aging men. The AMS scale grades the response of an individual to 17 questions covering sexual, psychological, and somato-vegetative aspects, with a minimum total score of 17 and maximum of 85. Responses were graded as normal (if the total score was below 27), mild (27–36), moderate (37–49), or severe (≥50).

However, one must remember that they are *not* diagnostic tools for androgen deficiency. In a couple of screening tests to detect men with androgen deficiency, arbitrarily defined as TT <13.8 nmol/L, it returned poor degrees of sensitivity and specificity, ranging only between 50 and 75 % (Kratzik et al. 2005).

Nevertheless, the AMS scale is a useful tool to gauge the impact of symptoms on an individual's quality of life, which may be used as justification for starting someone with low serum testosterone levels on androgen therapy. At the same time, it can track quite well the response of an individual to androgen therapy.

The severity of erectile dysfunction may be assessed using the modified International Index of Erectile Function (IIEF-5), comprising five questions with graded responses. Erectile dysfunction is graded as none if the score was 22–25, mild (17–21), mild-to-moderate ED (12–16), moderate ED (8–11), or severe ED (5–7). Again, the scores do not correlate with serum testosterone concentrations.

Reference Ranges

Most clinicians are used to the idea of fixed and established reference ranges for a wide variety of laboratory investigations, which provide easy means of making diagnoses. Unfortunately, in the case of androgen deficiency, the situation is far from being straightforward. Various methods of testosterone measurement exist, most of which do not fit the ideal, which should be inexpensive, easy to perform, widely available, accurate, and reproducible.

To date, serum total testosterone is the most widely recommended assay to be used in screening for androgen deficiency, being easily available and relatively inexpensive (Bhasin et al. 2006). Most laboratories quote a wide reference range of between 10 and 34 nmol/L, but as it is well established that serum testosterone concentrations fall with increasing age, it is clear that reference ranges must be age specific. However, to date, this is yet to be determined.

Total testosterone has its limitations when used in the context of age-related androgen deficiency in healthy males. This is because the serum concentration of sex hormone-binding globulin (SHBG) rises with increasing age. Since about 50 % of testosterone is bound to SHBG, any decline in testosterone may be masked by the higher levels of SHBG. This observation has been reported in population studies, where mean values of serum total testosterone did not show a declining trend across age groups (Li et al. 2005). The author's own experience with self-referred men seen at a men's health clinic has also been similar. Clearly, any situation affecting SHBG concentrations will have an impact on serum total testosterone concentrations as well. Hypogonadism itself may also cause levels of SHBG to be elevated, as may hyperthyroidism, cirrhosis, and anticonvulsant usage. Conversely, hypothyroidism, obesity, nephrotic syndrome, and androgen therapy may lower SHBG. Moreover, it has been reported that healthy men above 40 years old may have serum total testosterone as low as 7.4 nmol/L (Boyce et al. 2004). Should such men be considered androgen deficient, when they are otherwise well and asymptomatic? It, in fact, suggests that perhaps the lower limit of the normal reference range, instead of 10 nmol/L, should be lowered by another 3–4 nmol/L.

As the biological activity of testosterone largely resides with the tiny unbound fraction of free testosterone, the latter should, logically and preferably, be the measurement of choice in assessing androgen status, in the same vein as the utility of free thyroxine, instead of total thyroxine, in assessing thyroid status. Indeed, free testosterone, obtained either through measurement by equilibrium dialysis or calculated (online calculator available at http://www.issam.ch/freetesto.htm) using validated formula, (Vermeulen et al. 1999) does show a progressive linear decline with age (Li et al. 2005). One must remember to avoid using direct (analog) assays of free testosterone, which is poor in accuracy, with wide error margins of 40–80 % (Rosner et al. 2007).

The only drawback to using free testosterone is the lack of established reference ranges. Nevertheless, data is emerging that provides useful guidance. In an epidemiological study of 1,080 Chinese males (Li et al. 2005) (see Table 4.1), the median free testosterone for men younger than 50 years was at least 370 pmol/L, declining to 350 and 300 pmol/L for men aged 60–70 years and above 70 years, respectively. The 10th percentile of free testosterone in the same age categories was 225, 215, and 190 pmol/L.

From a cohort of self-referred, nondiabetic, relatively healthy Singaporean (predominantly Chinese) males ($N=201$) who were seen at the author's Men's Health clinic, the mean free testosterone for men in the same age categories was 328 pmol/L (95 % C.I. 301–354 pmol/L), 313 (297–329) pmol/L, and 273 (257–290) pmol/L, respectively. The 10th percentile in these age categories was 232, 208, and 181 pmol/L, respectively.

As one can see, the range of values of free testosterone between these two very different cohorts is fairly similar for subjects within the same age groups, especially for the lowest decile of values. This indicates that these values of free testosterone at the 10th percentile are likely to be good estimates of what is considered testosterone deficiency, specific for age.

Table 4.1 Age range and testosterone levels

	Total testosterone (nmol/L)		Calculated free testosterone (pmol/L)	
Age group (year)	Li et al. (2005) 10th percentile 90th percentile	Chen (CGH 2009)[a] 10th percentile 90th percentile	Li et al. (2005) 10th percentile 90th percentile	Chen (CGH 2009)[a] 10th percentile 90th percentile
Below 50	8.78	9.31	286	232
	32.93	23.23	587	461
50–59	11.43	9.45	225	208
	29.53	23.00	493	413
Above 60	13.88	9.66	215	181
	31.33	22.3	482	359

[a]Unpublished data from Men's Health and Andropause Clinic, Changi General Hospital

When all 201 subjects in the author's cohort were analyzed, the 50th, 25th, and 10th percentiles of free testosterone were found to be 297, 258, and 206 pmol/L, respectively. To pick convenient arbitrary cutoffs, these suggest that men with free testosterone above 300 pmol/L are androgen replete, while those with values just around, or below, 200 pmol/L are androgen deficient. This would be consistent with an earlier proposal by Vermeulen that free testosterone below 225 pmol/L (being 2SD below young adult mean) be used as a guide for diagnosing late-onset hypogonadism (Vermeulen 2005). Men with free testosterone below 250 pmol/L are likely to be androgen deficient, as they belong to the lowest quartile, and this level of free testosterone falls even below the lower limit of the 95 % confidence interval for older men above 60 years of age.

Is There Any Correlation Between Androgen Levels and Symptomatology?

It has been demonstrated, in a study of 434 men aged 50–86 years, that the prevalence of symptoms increases with decreasing testosterone concentrations (Zitzmann et al. 2006). Loss of libido and loss of vigor appear to be the earliest symptoms when serum testosterone concentration dips below 15 nmol/L. In fact, these symptoms carried a sensitivity of 82–88 % in detecting androgen deficiency. At levels below 10 nmol/L, depression, poorer mental concentrating ability, and sleep disturbances begin to surface. Hot flushes and erectile dysfunction are common complaints at levels below 8 nmol/L, and these two symptoms carried a fairly high specificity of 83–86 % for androgen deficiency.

Given this, it would seem logical to expect a correlation between the *degree of severity* of symptoms and androgen levels. As mentioned earlier, the AMS scale may be used to quantify symptom severity. However, it has been consistently shown that the AMS scale *does not* correlate with serum total or free testosterone concentrations (T'Sjoen et al. 2003). The author's own analysis on self-referred males, by their nature more likely to be androgen deficient, also revealed a total lack of correlation.

This is because different individuals possess different thresholds of androgen deficiency (Kelleher et al. 2004). A person may begin to experience symptoms of androgen deficiency at a total testosterone of, say, 12 nmol/L, whereas another individual may only be symptomatic at levels below 8 nmol/L. This also explains why it is not quite possible to set a definite cutoff value of serum testosterone to define androgen deficiency, due to the wide degree of interindividual variation.

Diagnosing Androgen Deficiency

Androgen deficiency is a clinical syndrome where symptoms play an important role in diagnosis. In general, diagnosing hormonal deficiency involves demonstrating clinical features of hormonal deficiency and proving, beyond doubt, that serum hormone concentrations are below the normal reference range.

Obviously, the main objectives of detecting hormonal deficiency are to reverse its undesirable effects on bodily systems, minimize or eliminate symptoms, and improve quality of life, by way of offering hormonal replacement therapy. Androgen replacement therapy (ART) in men with true androgen deficiency can readily lead to reversal of symptoms and improved body composition, strength, physical performance, sexual function, and bone mineral density, which translates into better overall quality of life. Outcome studies of ART on insulin resistance are equivocal, while no data is available yet on mortality outcome.

Any diagnostic criteria employed should serve not just for the detection of androgen deficiency but, more importantly, identify men who will benefit most from androgen replacement therapy (ART), from those in whom ART is unlikely to produce benefit. After all, ART is not free from risks. It makes sense to ensure that only the appropriate patients are selected in order to maximize benefit-to-risk ratio. Moreover, it is clear that the effects of ART are dependent on baseline testosterone levels – the lower the level of pretreatment testosterone, the greater the benefit (Snyder et al. 1999a, b).

Diagnosing True Androgen Deficiency

It is widely accepted that an early-morning (before 10:00 a.m.) serum total testosterone concentration below 10.4 nmol/L (300 ng/dL) on two separate occasions, in the presence of symptoms, is diagnostic of true androgen deficiency, regardless of age (Bhasin et al. 2006). Some adopt an even stricter criterion. The Australian consensus defines androgen deficiency as a morning total testosterone of less than 8.0 nmol/L (Conway et al. 2000). The lower cutoff helps to avoid the controversy in males with total testosterone just slightly below 10 nmol/L but who are, otherwise, asymptomatic. Generally, the diagnosis is quite straightforward in cases of clear-cut androgen deficiency, where androgen levels are extremely low and clinical signs of androgen deficiency are present.

Diagnosing Age-Related Relative Androgen Deficiency (Andropause)

The difficulty arises with diagnosing age-related relative androgen deficiency in older males (or andropause). Based on the current knowledge presented above, certain things are clear:

- No single symptom is pathognomonic of androgen deficiency. Rather, a symptom complex should be recognized.
- Free testosterone, probably the calculated form, is the measurement of choice. The direct (analog) assay is to be avoided.
- Taking into account that testosterone declines with age, as well as the wide variation in threshold for testosterone deficiency between individuals, a one-size-fits-all

cutoff value is not feasible. Rather, a level of free testosterone that is *inappropriately low for age* should be utilized.

- Nevertheless, serum-free testosterone concentrations below 250 pmol/L do appear to warrant consideration of androgen deficiency, while levels below 200 pmol/L are almost certainly deficient.

But not all such older men with lowish testosterone experience significant symptoms. In fact, only about 30–40 % of men do, while the remainder is relatively asymptomatic and healthy. Clearly, to make a diagnosis of andropause based on androgen levels alone is inappropriate. The severity of symptoms needs to be taken into consideration as well. After all, the whole point of diagnosing such individuals is to reverse symptoms and improve quality of life through ART, with minimal risks. To be successful, it is imperative that only appropriate individuals with good benefit-to-risk ratio are selected.

Therefore, with these considerations in mind, the author feels that the selection criteria require:

1. *Presence of significant symptoms* of at least moderate severity (arbitrarily defined as IIEF-5 <17 and/or AMS ≥50)
2. *Serum-free testosterone below 250 pmol/L or inappropriately low for age*

Suggested Workflow

For any male who complains of symptoms suggestive of androgen deficiency, the following initial assessment is recommended:

- Quantify his symptoms using both the AMS and IIEF-5 questionnaires.
- Measure blood pressure, waist circumference, and body mass index (BMI).
- Obtain early-morning blood samples for total testosterone, SHBG, luteinizing hormone (LH), follicle-stimulating hormone (FSH), and albumin. Calculate free testosterone.
- Include metabolic screen: obtain fasting lipid profile and fasting plasma glucose.

Men with serum total testosterone exceeding 14 nmol/L (400 ng/dL) are most probably normal. Their calculated free testosterone should easily exceed 300 pmol/L.

On the other hand, men with total testosterone below 10.4 nmol/L (300 ng/dL), or preferably below 8.0 nmol/L (230 ng/dL) to be even more definite, may be considered androgen deficient. Their calculated free testosterone (cFT) should be below 250 pmol/L and is likely to be even much lower. Before proceeding to offer ART, take a look at the LH/FSH values. If they appear to be inappropriately normal, or low, an MRI scan of the pituitary gland is mandatory to exclude any pituitary tumor. ART is contraindicated unless the tumor has been surgically resected.

For the group of men with inconclusive total testosterone values between 10 and 14 nmol/L (or 8–14 if a lower cutoff is used), the author adopts the following options:

- cFT <250 pmol/L with symptoms ⇒ offer ART
- cFT <250 pmol/L but asymptomatic ⇒ withhold treatment unless there are compelling reasons, e.g., osteoporosis
- cFT 250–300 pmol/L with significant symptoms ⇒ offer trial of ART
- cFT 250–300 pmol/L with only minimal symptoms ⇒ withhold ART
- cFT >300 pmol/L ⇒ normal (total testosterone may have been misleadingly low because of low SHBG)

The Implications of Andropause

It is prudent, at this stage, to remember that age-related relative androgen deficiency is somewhat different from true androgen deficiency, as testosterone concentrations in such men are only considered low for age, without being absolutely deficient. As mentioned earlier, not all older men with lowish testosterone are symptomatic. So, based on the arbitrary diagnostic criteria suggested above, what are the clinical implications of being labeled as having andropause?

Based on analysis of the author's cohort of self-referred, nondiabetic men ($n=187$), andropausal men ($n=66$) had significantly greater waist circumference and body mass index. Naturally, they also have significantly lower levels of total and free testosterone as well as lower IIEF-5 and AMS scores. However, no significant difference was found between andropausal and non-andropausal men for age, blood pressure, cholesterol components, and fasting glucose. Via logistic regression, the variables most likely to predict diagnosis of andropause were age, level of calculated free testosterone, and values of IIEF-5 and AMS somato-vegetative subscale.

The results indicate clearly that andropause is primarily a quality of life issue. Even though androgen deficiency has been linked with higher metabolic and cardiovascular risks, andropause does not identify such individuals. The onus, therefore, lies with the attending physician to conduct a metabolic screen for men with androgen deficiency on a case-by-case basis.

References

Bhasin S, Cunningham GR, Hayes FJ, Matsumoto AM, Snyder PJ, Swerdloff RS, Montori VM. Testosterone therapy in adult men with androgen deficiency syndromes: an endocrine society clinical practice guideline. J Clin Endocrinol Metab. 2006;91(6):1995–2010.

Boyce MJ, Baisley KJ, Clark EV, Warrington SJ. Are published normal ranges of serum testosterone too high? Results of a cross-sectional survey of serum testosterone and luteinizing hormone in healthy men. BJU Int. 2004;94(6):881–5.

Chen RY, Wittert GA, Andrews GR. Relative androgen deficiency in relation to obesity and metabolic status in older men. Diabetes Obes Metab. 2006;8(4):429–35.

Conway AJ, Handelsman DJ, Lording DW, Stuckey B, Zajac JD. Use, misuse and abuse of androgens The Endocrine Society of Australia consensus guidelines for androgen prescribing. Med J Aust. 2000;172(5):220–4. Erratum in: Med J Aust 2000 Apr 3;172(7):334.

Kelleher S, Conway AJ, Handelsman DJ. Blood testosterone threshold for androgen deficiency symptoms. J Clin Endocrinol Metab. 2004;89(8):3813–7.

Kratzik C, Heinemann LA, Saad F, Thai DM, Rücklinger E. Composite screener for androgen deficiency related to the Aging Males' Symptoms scale. Aging Male. 2005;8(3–4):157–61.

Laaksonen DE, Niskanen L, Punnonen K, Nyyssönen K, Tuomainen TP, Salonen R, Rauramaa R, Salonen JT. Sex hormones, inflammation and the metabolic syndrome: a population-based study. Eur J Endocrinol. 2003;149(6):601–8.

Laughlin GA, Barrett-Connor E, Bergstrom J. Low serum testosterone and mortality in older men. J Clin Endocrinol Metab. 2008;93(1):68–75.

Li JY, Li XY, Li M, Zhang GK, Ma FL, Liu ZM, Zhang NY, Meng P. Decline of serum levels of free testosterone in aging healthy Chinese men. Aging Male. 2005;8(3–4):203–6.

Rosner W, Auchus RJ, Azziz R, Sluss PM, Raff H. Position statement: utility, limitations, and pitfalls in measuring testosterone: an Endocrine Society position statement. J Clin Endocrinol Metab. 2007;92(2):405–13.

Snyder PJ, Peachey H, Hannoush P, Berlin JA, Loh L, Lenrow DA, Holmes JH, Dlewati A, Santanna J, Rosen CJ, Strom BL. Effect of testosterone treatment on body composition and muscle strength in men over 65 years of age. J Clin Endocrinol Metab. 1999a;84(8):2647–53.

Snyder PJ, Peachey H, Hannoush P, Berlin JA, Loh L, Holmes JH, Dlewati A, Staley J, Santanna J, Kapoor SC, Attie MF, Haddad Jr JG, Strom BL. Effect of testosterone treatment on bone mineral density in men over 65 years of age. J Clin Endocrinol Metab. 1999b;84(6):1966–72.

Stellato RK, Feldman HA, Hamdy O, Horton ES, McKinlay JB. Testosterone, sex hormone-binding globulin, and the development of type 2 diabetes in middle-aged men: prospective results from the Massachusetts male aging study. Diabetes Care. 2000;23(4):490–4.

T'Sjoen G, Feyen E, De Kuyper P, Comhaire F, Kaufman JM. Self-referred patients in an aging male clinic: much more than androgen deficiency alone. Aging Male. 2003;6(3):157–65.

Vermeulen A. Hormonal cut-offs of partial androgen deficiency: a survey of androgen assays. J Endocrinol Invest. 2005;28(3 Suppl):28–31.

Vermeulen A, Verdonck L, Kaufman JM. A critical evaluation of simple methods for the estimation of free testosterone in serum. J Clin Endocrinol Metab. 1999;84(10):3666–72.

Zitzmann M, Faber S, Nieschlag E. Association of specific symptoms and metabolic risks with serum testosterone in older men. J Clin Endocrinol Metab. 2006;91(11):4335–43.

Chapter 5
Testosterone Preparations for Treatment of Hypogonadal Men

Louis Gooren

Three approaches have been used to make testosterone therapeutically effective: (1) routes of administration, (2) esterification in the 17β-position, and (3) chemical modification of the molecule or a combination of approaches. In clinical practice, particularly in the perception of the patient, the route of administration is most relevant and is used to categorize the preparations described here (see Table 5.1).

Oral Preparations

Alkylated derivatives of testosterone including methyltestosterone, mesterolone, and fluoxymesterone are administered orally or sublingually. They are metabolized by the liver, like natural testosterone, but more slowly, and, like testosterone, interact directly with androgen receptors. The prolonged use (especially the 17α-alkylated androgens) has been associated with hepatotoxicity including hepatocellular adenoma, cholestatic jaundice, and hemorrhagic liver cysts, and their use is obsolete now. Mesterolone is safe but its androgenic potency is limited.

Oral Testosterone Undecanoate

Testosterone undecanoate (TU) is esterified testosterone dissolved in oil and encapsulated in soft gelatin. Of the 40 mg capsules, 63 % (25 mg) is testosterone. After ingestion, for a portion of around 5 % of the administered dose, the route of absorption from

L. Gooren, M.D., Ph.D.
Department of Endocrinology, Free University of Amsterdam, Amsterdam, the Netherlands

H.T. Naval Medical School, Surabaya, Indonesia
e-mail: louisjgooren@gmail.com

P.H.C. Lim (ed.), *Men's Health*,
DOI 10.1007/978-1-4471-4766-4_5, © Springer-Verlag London 2013

Table 5.1 Pharmacological aspects of different ways of testosterone administration

	Normal T/24 h	Normal E2	Normal DHT	Convenience	Dose flexibility	Satisfactory
Mesterolone	–	–	–	+	+	–
Oral TU	±	+	±	+	+	±
Transbuccal T	+	+	+	+	+	+
Sublingual T	+	+	+	+	+	+
Reservoir patch	+	+	+	+	–	+
T gel	+	+	+	+	+	++
T implants	+	+	+	+	±	++
Injectable T	–	±	±	±	–	±
Injectable TU	+	+	+	+	–	++
DHT gel	–	–	–	+	+	±

the gastrointestinal tract is shifted to the thoracic duct, avoiding a first pass through the liver and subsequent metabolism of testosterone. The dosing is, as a rule, two times 80 mg/day. For its adequate absorption from the gastrointestinal tract, it is essential that oral TU is taken with a meal that contains at least 18 g of dietary fat. It results in fluctuating serum testosterone levels. With a dose of 120–240 mg (3–6 capsules) per day, over 80 % of hypogonadal men showed plasma testosterone levels in the low normal range.

Transbuccal Testosterone Adminstration

Transbuccal administration of testosterone provides a means of oral administration of testosterone. It is marketed as a biopellet to be pressed on the gum above the incisor tooth. The resorption of testosterone through the oral mucosa bypasses intestinal absorption and subsequent hepatic inactivation of testosterone. Treatment with testosterone buccal system, (Striant®), 30 mg twice daily, generated serum testosterone in the normal range of 92.3 % patients. The effects of buccal testosterone on sexual functioning were comparable to those of parenteral testosterone enanthate.

Sublingual Testosterone Administration

Sublingual application of testosterone has been tested with the inclusion of the hydrophobic testosterone molecule with 2-hydroxypropyl-β-cyclodextrin (HPBCD). HPBCD enhances testosterone solubility and absorption, but HPBCD itself is not absorbed. Effects on sexual behavior are comparable to those of parenteral administration of 200 mg testosterone enanthate every 20 days.

Transdermal Preparations

Testosterone can be delivered to the circulation through the intact skin, both genital and nongenital. Transdermal administration delivers testosterone at a controlled rate into the systemic circulation, avoiding hepatic first pass and reproducing the diurnal rhythm of testosterone secretion, without the peak and trough levels observed in long-acting testosterone injections. Scrotal patches have fallen out of use.

Non-scrotal Testosterone Patch

These patches have a reservoir containing testosterone with a permeation-enhancing vehicle and gelling agents. Clinical efficacy is as good as with conventional testosterone ester injections. Despite being pharmacokinetically and clinically satisfactory, there are adverse effects such as local skin reactions.

Testosterone Gel

Testosterone gel is used for replacement therapy. Testosterone gel is hydroalcoholic, 1 % (10 mg testosterone per gram gel), and administered between 5 and 10 g of gel a day, amounting to 50 and 100 mg testosterone, and 9–14 % of the testosterone administered is bioavailable. The pharmacokinetics of testosterone gel has been extensively studied, and serum testosterone levels remain steadily in the middle-to-upper range of normal. The formulation of the testosterone gel allows easy dose adjustments (50–75–100 mg testosterone gel).

The safety profile and clinical efficacy of transdermal testosterone gel on various androgen-dependent target organ systems are very good. Skin irritation has been noted in 5.5 % of patients. Transfer from one person to another has been found but appears no great problem in general when precautions are observed. Skin contact should be avoided at least for the first hour after application.

Parenteral Preparations

Testosterone Implants

Subdermal pellet implantation was among the earliest effective treatment modalities for clinical use of testosterone and has become an established and inexpensive form of androgen replacement. Several reports have outlined its desirable pharmacological properties, but there may be complications, such as infection and extrusion.

Testosterone Esters

The most commonly used forms of ART include 17β-hydroxyl esters of testosterone administered with slow-release, oil-based vehicles. Commonly used intramuscular injectable testosterone esters are testosterone enanthate and cypionate.

Testosterone enanthate is one of the most widely used intramuscular testosterone ester. At a dose of 200–250 mg, the optimal injection interval is 2–3 weeks, but peak and through values are clearly above and below the normal range. Other testosterone esters are testosterone cypionate and testosterone cyclohexanocarboxylate. The pharmacokinetics of these testosterone esters is very similar to that of testosterone enanthate. Administration of 200 mg every 2 weeks provides an acceptable form of testosterone replacement.

Several commercially available testosterone preparations contain a number of short- and longer-acting testosterone esters aiming to deliver more even serum testosterone levels. Pharmacokinetic studies of these preparations show that this goal is not achieved. The peak values are higher than in single testosterone ester preparations, and resulting plasma testosterone levels show even larger fluctuations. So, most intramuscular preparations of testosterone esters are not ideal. With the most commonly used testosterone esters, a maximum concentration follows approximately 72 h after injection. Testosterone levels slowly diminish during the following 10–14 days showing an exponential decline of serum testosterone levels reaching baseline at approximately day 21. As a result the testosterone levels before the next injection are low. The profile of testosterone levels may be accompanied by disturbing fluctuations in sexual function, energy level, and mood. High postinjection levels of testosterone predispose the patient to acne and polycythemia, and elevated estradiol predisposes to gynecomastia. In some patients, injections may be associated with bleeding or bruising. However, these long-acting testosterone preparations have long time been the mainstay of testosterone treatment, and they are the most cost-effective methods, with administration of 200–400 mg every 2–4 weeks. The 200 mg injection will maintain normal testosterone for approximately 2 weeks, while 300 mg doses are required for eugonadal ranges for approximately 3 weeks.

Intramuscular Testosterone Undecanaote

Parenteral testosterone undecanoate (TU) is a new treatment modality for androgen therapy. The pharmacological principle of TU is the same as for other cleavable T fatty acid esters mentioned above. The much longer side chain of undecanoic acid with 11 carbon atoms permits considerably longer injection intervals of 10–13 weeks. At the same time, the supra- or sub-physiological serum T levels, so characteristic of the traditional T esters, are not observed.

Several studies have documented its use in hypogonadal men. Its attraction lies in the long duration of action. After adequate loading with injections at the beginning and after 6 weeks, most patients are well substituted with an administration every 12 weeks. Further, the resulting plasma testosterone levels are almost always in the physiological range, so the so-called roller coaster effect is rarely experienced by patients. Also, side effects of supraphysiological testosterone levels, such as polycythemia, are only rarely observed. There is now long-term experience up to more than 8–10 years with TU. Individual dosing ranged from 10 to 14 weeks, but exceptions to this rule, with complaints of testosterone deficiency after 6 weeks, have been observed. Serum trough levels of T, measured immediately before the new injection, are generally within the low normal range, indicating sufficient substitution over the total injection interval. In contrast to short-acting T esters, sensations of fluctuations in androgen serum concentrations are rarely observed. If this is the case, it occurs during the last 2 weeks before the next injection, indicating loss of androgenic psychotropic effects. Individualization of the TU therapy is recommended. If the T serum concentration before the 4th injection lies between 10 and 15 nmol/L, then the injection interval should be every 12 weeks. Should the T serum concentration at this time be lower than10 nmol/L, then the injection interval is shortened to every 10 weeks. If the T level is greater than 15 nmol/L, then the injection interval should be extended to every 14 weeks. Additionally, clinical symptoms should be taken into consideration to optimally adjust injection intervals with TU therapy. The loading dose of TU achieved by the first two injections with an interval of 6 weeks is also recommended for patients who are being transferred from short-acting testosterone injections (e.g., testosterone enanthate 250 mg) to treatment with long-acting TU.

In short, after two loading doses of 1,000 mg TU at 0 and 6 weeks, repeated injections at 12-week intervals are sufficient to maintain testosterone levels in the reference range of eugonadal men.

It has been argued that this preparation is less suitable for initiation of testosterone treatment of aging men. It is thought that the long duration of action might constitute a problem in case an intercurrent prostate malignancy will be diagnosed. Experienced urologists, however, reason that the delay between diagnosing prostate cancer and its treatment is usually much longer than 12 weeks, without an adverse effect on the outcome. In addition, current recommendations for administration of T to elderly men advocate initial follow-up at 3-month intervals for the first year, which fits very well into the schedule of TU injections. In the hypothetical case that a tumor is discovered, further treatment should be discontinued and the use of an antiandrogen may be considered. So, certainly after the first uneventful year of androgen administration, it seems reasonable to administer long-acting testosterone preparations to elderly men.

Alternative Methods

Androgen Replacement with 5α-Reduced Testosterone: 5α-Dihydrotestosterone

The effects of testosterone are mediated directly as testosterone or after conversion to either 5α-dihydrotestosterone (DHT) or estradiol locally in target tissues. The reduction of testosterone to DHT is an amplification mechanism of the androgenizing effects of testosterone. DHT binds to the same receptor as testosterone, but its receptor binding is stronger, resulting in a considerable higher biopotency than testosterone itself. DHT, as opposed to testosterone, cannot be aromatized to estradiol and acts, therefore, as a pure androgen. In certain clinical conditions, a pure androgen might have advantages over aromatizable testosterone, such as cases of a microphallus, hypogonadal men with a susceptibility to gynecomastia or constitutionally delayed puberty in boys. Estrogens are pivotal in closure of the epiphyses in puberty, and a non-aromatizable androgen might allow some extra gain in height by slowing the closure of the pubertal epiphyses. Studies of DHT administration to hypogonadal men show that DHT maintains sex characteristics, increases muscle mass, and improves sexual functions without significant increases in prostate size.

Androgen Stimulation with Human Chorionic Gonadotrophin

Administration of testosterone has no role to play in men who have fertility problems. If they are hypogonadal, their testosterone levels can be raised with parenteral administration of human chorionic gonadotrophin, 1,500 iU, two to three times per week. Apart from stimulation of testosterone, also plasma estradiol levels rise with the potential side effect of gynecomastia.

Chapter 6
Androgens, Use, Misuse, and Abuse

Louis Gooren

Androgens have a relatively long history of about 70 years since their characterization in the mid-1930s. This contribution tries to define and optimize their appropriate clinical use, to minimize their misuse, and to avoid their abuse.

Use for Appropriate Indications

Testosterone is used clinically in two different ways: as androgen replacement therapy and as pharmacological androgen therapy.

Androgen replacement therapy aims to replicate, as closely as possible, androgen exposure of all androgen-dependent tissues of the body with doses that mimic as close as possible endogenous testosterone production of the eugonadal male. Pharmacological androgen therapy uses androgens like any other chemical drug, judged by the standards of efficacy for their purpose and their safety.

1. Androgen deficiency or hypogonadism is the principal indication for androgen replacement therapy. In androgen replacement therapy, testosterone is used at doses designed to reproduce endogenous blood testosterone levels and aims to achieve physiological exposure of androgen-dependent tissues/organs to testosterone. The more optimal this goal is attained, the better the health outcomes of androgen replacement in testosterone-deficient men. It will enhance energy, motivation, and endurance and it will produce/restore structural and functional deficits in muscle,

This contribution has heavily drawn from the article by Handelsman DJ. Testosterone: use, misuse and abuse. Med J Aust. 2006;185(8):436–9. Review.

L. Gooren, M.D., Ph.D.
Department of Endocrinology, Free University of Amsterdam, Amsterdam, the Netherlands

H.T. Naval Medical School, Surabaya, Indonesia
e-mail: louisjgooren@gmail.com

P.H.C. Lim (ed.), *Men's Health*,
DOI 10.1007/978-1-4471-4766-4_6, © Springer-Verlag London 2013

bone, erythropoiesis and glucose/lipid metabolism, and psychosexual activity, therewith substantially improving quality of life. Specific time limited use includes delayed puberty and hypogonadal elderly men. Recent insight has shown that men have different but individually consistent blood testosterone thresholds for the biological actions of testosterone. This is due to properties of their genetic makeup of receptors of testosterone action. So, inevitably, there will be some degree of difference in the doses of testosterone needed for optimal androgen replacement treatment, but these differences should not be exaggerated. Recent studies indicate that many hypogonadal men are not (adequately) treated with testosterone. Often the hypogonadal state of these men (predominantly men with Klinefelter's syndrome) is not diagnosed since men undergo significantly fewer genital examinations compared to women. The consequence of this underdiagnosis of male hypogonadism is that not so few men have a suboptimal health state and lead unfulfilled lives.

2. Use in women: It is now widely believed that testosterone has also a role in female sexual desire. Hypoactive sexual desire disorder (HSDD; loss of desire that causes personal distress) is not uncommon, though estimated prevalences range between 8 and 50 %. Women with HSDD experience poor sexual self-image, feelings of unattractiveness, fear of disappointing their partners, depression, anxiety, and diminished quality of life. Sometimes men and women report a discrepancy between their own and their partner's sexual desire, and they often have lower relationship satisfaction. Individuals in sexually inactive marriages report less marital happiness. Thus, HSDD merits attention. Counseling and general sex education may be helpful. But often postmenopausal women continue to experience HSDD despite good clinical care. There are now a series of randomized controlled trials evaluating the efficacy and safety of transdermal testosterone patch therapy in postmenopausal women with HSDD. Studies have shown that women treated with a patch delivering 300 μg of testosterone per day were more likely to report a meaningful benefit than women receiving placebo, with more than 85 % of those reporting a benefit wishing to continue treatment. Side effects are increased sexual hair growth and enlargement of the clitoris. The effects of androgens on breast cancer development are uncertain.
3. Pharmacological androgen therapy aims not to mimic androgen testosterone production but is used for its salutary effects in men with chronic diseases in an attempt to change the course of that disease and to improve quality of life. A number of its uses have been overtaken by newer drugs. Examples are:

   (a) Anemia due to bone marrow failure, stimulating erythropoiesis and reducing the need for blood transfusion.
   (b) Chronic respiratory failure to improve strength of chest musculature.
   (c) Chronic cardiac failure to improve the pump function of the heart.
   (d) Steroid-dependent autoimmune disease. Testosterone may counteract the catabolic effects of corticosteroids.
   (e) Muscle wasting as in AIDS.
   (f) Preventing attacks of hereditary angioedema or urticaria.
   (g) Still undergoing clinical testing is the use of androgens for rehabilitation of burns and muscle wasting with major surgery such as hip replacement.

Misuse: Prescription of Androgen for Unproven Indications

A frequent misuse of androgens is in men with fertility problems and stems from lack of insight into the hormonal regulation of spermatogenesis. Spermatogenesis is dependent on the pituitary hormone FSH and on high local concentration of testosterone in the testis. Testicular levels of testosterone required for spermatogenesis cannot be attained with exogenous testosterone administration. Exogenous testosterone is rather counterproductive. Testosterone (after its conversion to estradiol) suppresses FSH, necessary for initiation of spermatogenesis, and also LH, the hormone for synthesis of testicular testosterone production providing the high local levels of testosterone required for the later stages of spermatogenesis. There is no exception to the rule that testosterone administration has no role in treating men with fertility problems.

It is difficult to draw a firm line between prudent use of testosterone, a concern with so many men not receiving adequate androgen treatment, and an overprescription of testosterone to men with dubious indications for testosterone replacement. The indication for androgen replacement should be based on clinical signs of androgen deficiency supported by laboratory evidence of levels of testosterone below reference values. Particularly, in elderly men the clinical signs of androgen deficiency may not be as salient as in younger men. Also the laboratory diagnosis of testosterone deficiency has its pitfalls and problems (lack of standardization of methods of testosterone measurement). This issue is addressed in the section on laboratory diagnosis of testosterone deficiency.

Abuse: Nonmedical Indications

The most illustrious abuse of testosterone and its derivatives is their use to advance competition in sports, particularly power sports where greater muscle mass leads to greater strength, but they are also used in sports that require quick action and endurance to combat muscle fatigue. There are unscrupulous medical doctors who provide guidance to elite sportsmen and sportswomen in the use of androgens and other substances claimed to give a competitive edge. But for the larger part, preparations used have been illegally obtained. Their manufacture may be illicit or produced by unknown manufactures in countries with lax law enforcement regarding production and sale of drugs, and it is not rare that the chemical composition is totally different from what the label indicates. Their indication is sometimes veterinary use.

Much wider is the abuse of androgens in circles of body building by men who strive to have an intimidating muscularity and strength. Among these men there is a lot of folklore concerning androgen preparations. The provenance of the drugs is as above. Of late the use of anabolic steroids has not been limited to men: there are also female users.

Unfortunately, their use has been spread to many adolescents who are dissatisfied with their body image and hope for quick successes in building up muscles and strength so as to perform well in sports and have a competitive edge in finding a sexual partner.

Doctors may identify this abuse in men with an extraordinary degree of muscularity, excessive frequency of exercise in gyms, often with obsessive traits. Physically, there may be acne, gynecomastia, and testicular atrophy (as a result of suppression of FSH and subsequent atrophy of spermatogenetic epithelium). In case of use of derivatives of testosterone, endogenous testosterone levels will be low. It may take several months, even years, to recover from the suppression of endogenous LH and FSH produced by the drugs used. Therefore, it is sometimes difficult to break this cycle. Stopping of anabolic steroids will produce a state of low endogenous testosterone production with its negative psychological and sexual traits. Also fertility, requiring normal endogenous FSH and LH production, may be problematic. There is not much information how to guide men with serious abuse of anabolic steroids to terminating them.

Anabolic steroids can have effects that are akin to that of other drugs of abuse. Use of anabolic steroids is often associated with illicit use of other drugs of abuse, as well as physiological and behavioral consequences (including violence and aggression). Anabolic-androgenic steroids use may lead to addiction, dependence, and withdrawal effects so that use is often continued despite short- and long-term health risks. Anabolic steroids have receptor- and non-receptor-bound effects, but there is a lack of basic understanding of androgens' actions and their hedonic effects and their neurobiological mechanisms. It has been hypothesized that androgens may produce some of their positive hedonic effects by enhancing 3α-diol production, which, in turn, have actions at gamma-aminobutyric/benzodiazepine receptor complexes in the nucleus accumbens; the latter has synapses with dopaminergic neurons. Withdrawal of androgens may lead to a wide range of psychiatric manifestations.

Several organizations of medical professionals and legal systems prohibit now the prescription of substances for the above purposes. In some countries testosterone has become a controlled substance of which the prescription requires medical documentation of the indication for its use.

Bibliography

Achar S, Rostamian A, Narayan SM. Cardiac and metabolic effects of anabolic-androgenic steroid abuse on lipids, blood pressure, left ventricular dimensions, and rhythm. Am J Cardiol. 2010;106(6):893–901.

Arnold AM, Peralta JM, Thonney ML. Ontogeny of growth hormone, insulin-like growth factor-I, estradiol and cortisol in the growing lamb: effect of testosterone. J Endocrinol. 1996;150(3): 391–9.

Baggish AL, Weiner RB, Kanayama G, Hudson JI, Picard MH, Hutter Jr AM, et al. Long-term anabolic-androgenic steroid use is associated with left ventricular dysfunction. Circ Heart Fail. 2010;3(4):472–6.

Bahrke MS, Yesalis 3rd CE, Wright JE. Psychological and behavioural effects of endogenous testosterone levels and anabolic-androgenic steroids among males. A review. Sports Med. 1990;10(5):303–37.

Basaria S. Androgen abuse in athletes: detection and consequences. J Clin Endocrinol Metab. 2010;95(4):1533–43.

Basaria S, Wahlstrom JT, Dobs AS. Clinical review 138: anabolic-androgenic steroid therapy in the treatment of chronic diseases. J Clin Endocrinol Metab. 2001;86(11):5108–17.

Berger JR, Pall L, Hall CD, et al. Oxandrolone in AIDS-wasting myopathy. AIDS. 1996;10(14): 1657–62.

Berkow R, editor. The Merck manual of diagnosis and therapy. 15th ed. Rahway: Merck Sharp and Dohme Research Laboratories; 1987. p. 1208.

Birgner C, Kindlundh-Högberg AM, Alsiö J, et al. The anabolic androgenic steroid nandrolone decanoate affects mRNA expression of dopaminergic but not serotonergic receptors. Brain Res. 2008;1240:221–8.

Bucher, Berger, Fields-Gardner, et al. A prospective study on the safely and effect of nandrolone decanoate in HIV positive patients. Abstract of the 11th Conf. on AIDS. Vancouver. 1996.

Danhaive PA, Rousseau GG. Binding of glucocorticoid antagonists to androgen and glucocorticoid hormone receptors in rat skeletal muscle. J Steroid Biochem. 1986;24(2):481–7.

Demling R, De Santi L. Closure of the "non-healing wound" corresponds with correction of weight loss using the anabolic agent oxandrolone. Ostomy Wound Manage. 1998;44(10):58–62, 64, 66 passim.

Di Paolo M, Agozzino M, Toni C, et al. Sudden anabolic steroid abuse-related death in athletes. Int J Cardiol. 2007;114(1):114–7. Epub 2005 Dec 20.

Di Pasquale MG. Drug use and detection in amateur sports. Warkworth: MGD Press; 1984.

Dimick DF, Heron M, Baulieu EE, et al. A comparative study of the metabolic fate of testosterone, 17 alpha-methyl-testosterone. 19-nor-testosterone. 17 alpha-methyl-19-nor-testosterone and 17 alpha-methylestr-5(10)-ene-17 beta-ol-3-one in normal males. Clin Chim Acta. 1961;6: 63–71.

Falanga V, Greenberg AS, Zhou L, et al. Stimulation of collagen synthesis by the anabolic steroid stanozolol. J Invest Dermatol. 1998;111(6):1193–7.

Ferreira IM, Verreschi IT, Nery LE, et al. The influence of 6 months of oral anabolic steroids on body mass and respiratory muscles in undernourished COPD patients. Chest. 1998;114(1): 19–28.

Fineschi V, Riezzo I, Centini F, et al. Sudden cardiac death during anabolic steroid abuse: morphologic and toxicologic findings in two fatal cases of bodybuilders. Int J Legal Med. 2007;121(1):48–53. Epub 2005 Nov 15.

Gaughan WJ, Liss KA, Dunn SR, et al. A 6-month study of low-dose recombinant human erythropoietin alone and in combination with androgens for the treatment of anemia in chronic hemodialysis patients. Am J Kidney Dis. 1997;30(4):495–500.

Gaul C, Morato T, Hayano M, et al. Biosynthesis of estrogens. Endocrinology. 1962;71:920–5.

Gold J, High HA, Li Y, et al. Safety and efficacy of nandrolone decanoate for treatment of wasting in patients with HIV infection. AIDS. 1996;10(7):745–52.

Graham MR, Evans P, Davies B, Baker JS. AAS, growth hormone, and insulin abuse: psychological and neuroendocrine effects. Ther Clin Risk Manag. 2008;4(3):587–97.

Johansen KL, Mulligan K, Schambelan M. Anabolic effects of nandrolone decanoate in patients receiving dialysis: a randomized controlled trial. JAMA. 1999;281(14):1275–81.

Kokkevi A, Fotiou A, Chileva A, et al. Daily exercise and anabolic steroids use in adolescents: a cross-national European study. Subst Use Misuse. 2008;43:2053–65.

Lau DH, Stiles MK, John B, et al. Atrial fibrillation and anabolic steroid abuse. Int J Cardiol. 2007;117(2):e86–7.

Mendenhall CL, Moritz TE, Roselle GA, et al. A study of oral nutritional support with oxandrolone in malnourished patients with alcoholic hepatitis: results of a Department of Veterans Affairs cooperative study. Hepatology. 1993;17(4):564–76.

Phillis BD, Abeywardena MY, Adams MJ, et al. Nandrolone potentiates arrhythmogenic effects of cardiac ischemia in the rat. Toxicol Sci. 2007;99(2):605–11. Epub 2007 Jul 25.

Rada RT, Kellner R, Winslow WW. Plasma testosterone and aggressive behavior. Psychosomatics. 1976;17(3):138–42.

Rosenfeld RL. Role of androgens in growth and development of the fetus, child, and adolescent. Adv Pediatr. 1972;19:171–213.

Samuels LT, Sellers DM, McCaulay CJ. The source of excess creatine following methyl testosterone. J Clin Endocrinol Metab. 1946;6:655–63.

Schols AM, Soeters PB, Mostert R, et al. Physiologic effects of nutritional support and anabolic steroids in patients with chronic obstructive pulmonary disease. A placebo-controlled randomized trial. Am J Respir Crit Care Med. 1995;152(4 Pt 1):1268–74.

Schwingel PA, Cotrim HP, Salles BR, Almeida CE, dos Santos Jr CR, Nachef B, et al. Anabolic-androgenic steroids: a possible new risk factor of toxicant-associated fatty liver disease. Liver Int. 2011;31(3):348–53.

Snyder PJ, Peachey H, Hannoush P, et al. Effect of testosterone treatment on bone mineral density in men over 65 years of age. J Clin Endocrinol Metab. 1999;84(6):1966–72.

Spungen AM, Grimm DR, Strakhan M, et al. Treatment with an anabolic agent is associated with improvement in respiratory function in persons with tetraplegia: a pilot study. Mt Sinai J Med. 1999;66(3):201–5.

Steele RE, Didato F, Steinetz BG. Relative importance of 5alpha reduction for the androgenic and LH-inhibiting activities of delta-4-3-ketosteroids. Steroids. 1977;29(3):331–48.

Strawford A, Barbieri T, Van Loan M, et al. Resistance exercise and supraphysiologic androgen therapy in eugonadal men with HIV-related weight loss: a randomized controlled trial. JAMA. 1999;281(14):1282–90.

Talih F, Fattal O, Malone Jr D. Anabolic steroid abuse: psychiatric and physical costs. Cleve Clin J Med. 2007;74(5):341–4, 346, 349–52.

Urban RJ, Bodenburg YH, Gilkison C, et al. Testosterone administration to elderly men increases skeletal muscle strength and protein synthesis. Am J Physiol. 1995;269(5 Pt 1):E820–6.

Vogel W, Klaiber EL, Broverman DM. A comparison of the antidepressant effects of a synthetic androgen (mesterolone) and amitriptyline in depressed men. J Clin Psychiatry. 1985;46(1): 6–8.

Wilson IC, Prange Jr AJ, Lara PP. Methyltestosterone with imipramine in men: conversion of depression to paranoid reaction. Am J Psychiatry. 1974;131(1):21–4.

Chapter 7
Testosterone Therapy, Prostate Safety, and Other Safety Issues

Ng Kok Kit

Testosterone replacement therapy has dramatically improved the quality of life of many men with late-onset hypogonadism. However, one concern that many doctors and patients have regarding this therapy is prostate safety. The main concern is the possible association with prostate cancer and minor concern with benign prostatic hyperplasia (BPH). As part of the natural history of the prostate, both the incidence and prevalence of both BPH and prostate cancer increase with aging men. In the natural scheme of things, testosterone level decreases with age. We were taught at medical school that prostate cancer and BPH are androgen dependent, and many doctors have great trepidation in giving the highly effective testosterone replacement therapy as a result of this. However, the current body of evidence generally sees no harm to the prostate in giving testosterone replacement therapy. There is no conclusive evidence (Roddam et al. 2008; Carpenter et al. 2008) that testosterone therapy increases the risk of prostate cancer or BPH.

History of Testosterone and Prostate Cancer

How did the association between testosterone and prostate cancer come about? In 1941, Huggins and Hodges (1941) showed that castration and estrogen treatment caused acid phosphatase levels (marker for metastatic prostate cancer) to decline in

Ng.K. Kit, MBBS (Singapore), FRCS (Glas), FRCS (Edin), FAMS (Urology)
Department of Urology, Changi General Hospital, Singapore, Singapore

Andropause and Men's Health Clinic, Changi General Hospital, Singapore, Singapore
e-mail: kok_kit_ng@cgh.com.sg

P.H.C. Lim (ed.), *Men's Health*,
DOI 10.1007/978-1-4471-4766-4_7,

men in metastatic prostate cancer. This has resulted in the use of androgen deprivation therapy as the mainstay for the treatment of metastatic prostate cancer. In addition to this, they showed that daily injection of testosterone propionate caused acid phosphatase levels to increase. However, this is found in only one subject, where the acid phosphatase level rose during 18 days of testosterone injection, but fluctuated widely before and afterward, resulting in the same peak levels 3 weeks after discontinuation of testosterone. Therefore, the original assertion that testosterone caused prostate cancer growth in untreated individuals were based on equivocal acid phosphatase levels in a single individual.

Contraindication to Testosterone Therapy

Who should not have testosterone therapy? There is evidence that testosterone can stimulate the growth and aggravate symptoms in men with locally advanced and metastatic prostate cancer. The largest series of exogenous testosterone in men with metastatic prostate cancer was reported by Fowler and Whitmore (1981), from Memorial Sloan-Kettering Cancer Center in New York. Sixty-seven men, all with history of bony metastases, received testosterone injections under various protocols, and unfavorable responses were noted, which included subjective symptoms, such as increased bone pain, or objective progression, including a rise in acid phosphatase.

Prostate Cancer in Men Receiving Testosterone Therapy

Does testosterone therapy lead to prostate cancer? According to a study by Gooren et al. (2007), the most frequently cited concern of physicians using testosterone therapy is that the treatment might induce prostate cancer. However, data assessing the relationship between the incidence of prostate cancer in men receiving testosterone therapy are sparse. The few case reports (Loughlin and Richie 1997; Gaylis et al. 2005; Jackson et al. 1989) and small retrospective studies have described the development of prostate cancer after testosterone therapy was initiated, but prostate biopsies were not performed prior to testosterone therapy. As prostate cancer is common in older men, the reported prostate cancer diagnoses could just be a coincidence rather than due to testosterone therapy itself. In addition, the number of men receiving testosterone therapy has increased greatly in recent years, and the reported number of prostate cancer cases after testosterone therapy appears to be too small to suggest a clear association.

Rhoden and Morgentaler reported on the incidence of prostate cancer in seven testosterone therapy trials (Rhoden and Morgentaler 2004), of which three were placebo controlled. Prostate cancer was detected in only 5 of the 461 evaluated men (1.1 %). A meta-analysis (Calof et al. 2005) was performed by Calof et al. on 19 double-blinded, randomized, placebo-controlled trials on testosterone therapy in men >45 years. No statistically significant greater rate of prostate cancer was recorded in testosterone-treated men than in men receiving placebo. In 2006, Marks et al. showed that testosterone therapy does not exert a deleterious effect on prostate. He randomized 44 men with late-onset hypogonadism to either parenteral testosterone or placebo for 6 months. Prostate biopsies were performed prior to randomization to rule out prostate cancer and to assess the prostate tissue levels of testosterone and DHT before testosterone therapy. Some 6 months after randomization, the patients underwent repeat biopsies. There were no significant changes in the intraprostatic levels of testosterone or DHT. Prostate volume was also not significantly changed by testosterone therapy. At repeat biopsy, small prostate cancer foci were found in four men of the placebo group versus two men of the testosterone arm.

Does testosterone therapy increase the risk of prostate cancer in men at increased risk of prostate cancer, such as those with prostatic intraepithelial neoplasia (PIN)? In a study by Rhoden and Morgentaler (2003), 20 hypogonadal men with biopsy-proven PIN were treated with testosterone therapy for 12 months, and their results were compared to 55 men without PIN. There was no significant difference in PSA responses between these two groups, and in follow-up, only a single prostate cancer was detected (in the PIN group).

In animal studies (Umekita et al. 1996; Chuu et al. 2005), it was shown that testosterone therapy suppressed prostate cancer growth and even to cause reversion from androgen-independent to androgen-dependent phenotypes. These experimental findings suggest that testosterone therapy may even be beneficial in certain prostate cancer types.

Testosterone Therapy After Definitive Treatment of Localized Prostate Cancer

Currently, the majority of prostate cancers diagnosed are localized. Treatment options for localized prostate cancer include radical prostatectomy, external beam radiotherapy, or interstitial brachytherapy. How about the use of testosterone therapy in patients who had their localized prostate cancer treated successfully and had clinical symptoms and signs of hypogonadism?

Traditionally, prostate cancer is an absolute contraindication for testosterone therapy. Recently, there are an increasing number of patients with localized prostate cancer, and many of these patients are treated successfully. Many of these patients also concomitantly have late-onset hypogonadism. There are few studies (Isbarn et al. 2009) on the use of testosterone therapy after successful definitive treatment. Five series (Agarwal and Oefelein 2005; Kaufman and Graydon 2004) with a small combined sample size ($n = 74$) have reported on the effect of testosterone therapy after radical prostatectomy. Of the 74 patients reported overall, only 1 (1.4 %) experienced biochemical recurrence after testosterone therapy. This particular patient had a high-grade cancer, which is an established risk factor for biochemical recurrence.

In patients with localized prostate cancer and who had undergone interstitial brachytherapy or external beam radiotherapy (EBRT), the question of testosterone therapy safety is even more intriguing because the prostate remains in situ. Studies done showed no biochemical recurrence in patients treated with brachytherapy (Sarosdy 2007) or EBRT (Davilla et al. 2008; Morales et al. 2009). However, it must be noted that all these studies of testosterone therapy in patients with treated prostate cancer are small series.

Testosterone Therapy and Benign Prostatic Hyperplasia

When men become older, there is a proliferation of the cells in the prostate gland, which results in the prostate gland becoming larger; this process is called benign prostatic hyperplasia (BPH). This causes various lower urinary tract symptoms (LUTS). But does testosterone therapy worsen BPH or LUTS? Currently, there is no compelling data to suggest that testosterone therapy exacerbates LUTS or promotes acute urinary retention. According to the ISSAM guidelines (Wang et al. 2009), severe LUTS evident by a high (>21) International Prostate Symptom Score (IPSS) due to BPH represent a relative contraindication, though evidence is weak. However, after successful treatment of lower urinary tract obstruction, this contraindication is no longer applicable.

Clinical Guidelines on Testosterone Therapy in Relation to Prostate Issue

Prior to Testosterone Therapy

Risk of prostate cancer assessed by:

- *Doing a digital rectal examination (DRE).*
  Look for prostate nodules.
- *Doing a serum prostate-specific antigen (PSA).*
  Pretreatment prostate ultrasound examinations or biopsies are not recommended as routine requirements.

However, if DRE or PSA are suspicious, then the patient should be referred to a urologist for assessment for prostate cancer.

Risk of LUTS is assessed by:

- *International Prostate Symptom Score (IPSS) questionnaire* (Table 7.1).
  If severe LUTS are detected (if IPSS >21), the patient may need to be treated for LUTS first before initiating testosterone therapy.

Table 7.1 International Prostate Symptom Score (IPSS)

Name: **Date:**

	Not at all	Less than 1 time in 5	Less than half the time	About half the time	More than half the time	Almost always	Your score
Incomplete emptying Over the past month, how often have you had a sensation of not emptying your bladder completely after you finish urinating?	0	1	2	3	4	5	
Frequency Over the past month, how often have you had to urinate again less than 2 h after you finished urinating?	0	1	2	3	4	5	
Intermittency Over the past month, how often have you found you stopped and started again several times when you urinated?	0	1	2	3	4	5	
Urgency Over the last month, how difficult have you found it to postpone urination?	0	1	2	3	4	5	
Weak stream Over the past month, how often have you had a weak urinary stream?	0	1	2	3	4	5	
Straining Over the past month, how often have you had to push or strain to begin urination?	0	1	2	3	4	5	

(continued)

Table 7.1 (continued)

	None	1 time	2 times	3 times	4 times	5 times or more	Your score
Nocturia Over the past month, many times did you most typically get up to urinate from the time you went to bed until the time you got up in the morning?	0	1	2	3	4	5	

Total IPSS score							

Quality of life due to urinary symptoms	**Delighted**	**Pleased**	**Mostly satisfied**	**Mixed – about equally**	**Mostly**	**Unhappy**	**Terrible**
If you were to spend the rest of your life with your urinary condition the way it is now, how would you feel about that?	0	1	2	3	4	5	6

Total score: 0–7 mildly symptomatic, 8–19 moderately symptomatic, 20–35 severely symptomatic

Monitoring During Testosterone Therapy

- *Do DRE and PSA every 3–6 months.*
  Patients should be monitored for prostate disease at 3–6 months, 12 months, and at least annually thereafter. Should the patient's prostate cancer risk be sufficiently high (suspicious finding on DRE or increased PSA), the patient should be referred to a urologist for transrectal ultrasound (TRUS) and biopsies of the prostate (Bhasin et al. 2003).

Testosterone Therapy for Men Successfully Treated for Prostate Cancer

Men successfully treated for prostate cancer and suffering from confirmed symptomatic hypogonadism are potential candidates for testosterone therapy after a prudent interval if there is no clinical or laboratory evidence of residual cancer. As long-term outcome data are not available, clinicians must exercise good clinical judgment together with adequate knowledge of advantages and drawbacks of testosterone therapy in this situation. The risks and benefits must be clearly discussed with and understood by the patient, and the follow-up must be particularly careful.

Other Safety Issues

Men with significant erythrocytosis (hematocrit >52 %), untreated obstructive sleep apnea, or untreated severe congestive heart failure should not be started on treatment (Calof et al. 2005) with testosterone without prior resolution of the comorbid condition.

Erythrocytosis can develop during testosterone treatment. Periodic hematological assessment is indicated (i.e., before treatment, then at 3–4 months and at 12 months in the first year of treatment, and annually thereafter). While it is not yet clear what critical threshold is desirable, dose adjustments and/or periodic phlebotomy may be necessary to keep hematocrit below 52–55 %.

References

Agarwal PK, Oefelein MG. Testosterone replacement therapy after primary treatment for prostate cancer. J Urol. 2005;173:533–6.

Bhasin S, Singh AB, Mac R, Carter B, Lee MI, Cunningham GR. Managing the risks of prostate disease during testosterone replacement therapy in older men: recommendations for a standardized monitoring plan. J Androl. 2003;24:299–311.

Calof OM, Singh AB, Lee ML, et al. Adverse events associated with testosterone replacement in middle-aged men: a meta-analysis of randomized, placebo-controlled trials. J Gerontol A Biol Sci Med Sci. 2005;60:1451–7.

Carpenter WR, Robinson WR, Godley PA. Getting over testosterone: postulating a fresh start for etiologic studies of prostate cancer. J Natl Cancer Inst. 2008;100:158–9.

Chuu CP, Hiipakka RA, Fukuchi J, Kokontis JM, Liao S. Androgen causes growth suppression and reversion of androgen-independent prostate cancer xenografts to an androgen-stimulated phenotype in athymic mice. Cancer Res. 2005;65:2082–4.

Davilla H, Arison C, Hall M, Salup R, Lockhart J, Carrion R. Analysis of the PSA response after testosterone supplementation in patients who previously received management for their localized prostate cancer. J Urol. 2008;179(Suppl):428, abstract 1247.

Fowler JE, Whitmore Jr WF. The response of metastatic adenocarcinoma of the prostate to exogenous testosterone. J Urol. 1981;126:372–5.

Gaylis FD, Lin DW, Ignatoff JM, Amling CL, Tutrone RF, Cosgrove DJ. Prostate cancer in men using testosterone supplementation. J Urol. 2005;174:534–8, discussion 538.

Gooren LJ, Behre HM, Saad F, Frank A, Schwerdt S. Diagnosing and treating testosterone deficiency in different parts of the world. Results from global market research. Aging Male. 2007;10:173–81.

Huggins C, Hodges CV. Studies on prostatic cancer, I: the effect of castration, of estrogen and of androgen injection on serum phosphatases in metastatic carcinoma of the prostate. Cancer Res. 1941;1:293–7.

Isbarn H, Pinthus JH, Marks LS, Montorsi F, Morales A, Morgentaler A, Schulman C. Testosterone and prostate cancer: revisiting old paradigms. Eur Urol. 2009;56:48–56.

Jackson JA, Waxman J, Spiekerman AM. Prostatic complications of testosterone replacement therapy. Arch Intern Med. 1989;149:2365–6.

Kaufman JM, Graydon RJ. Androgen replacement after curative radical prostatectomy for prostate cancer in hypogonadal men. J Urol. 2004;172:920–2.

Loughlin KR, Richie JP. Prostate cancer after exogenous testosterone treatment for impotence. J Urol. 1997;157:1845.

Morales A, Black AM, Emerson LE. Testosterone administration to men with testosterone deficiency syndrome after external beam radiotherapy for localized prostate cancer: preliminary observations. BJU Int. 2009;103:62–4.

Rhoden EL, Morgentaler A. Testosterone replacement therapy in hypogonadal men at high risk for prostate cancer: result of 1 year of treatment in men with prostatic intraepithelial neoplasia. J Urol. 2003;170:2348–51.

Rhoden EL, Morgentaler A. Risks of testosterone-replacement therapy and recommendations for monitoring. N Engl J Med. 2004;350:482–92.

Roddam AW, Allen NE, Appleby P, Key TJ. Endogenous sex hormones and prostate cancer: a collaborative analysis of 18 prospective studies. J Natl Cancer Inst. 2008;100:170–83.

Sarosdy MF. Testosterone replacement for hypogonadism after treatment of early prostate cancer with brachytherapy. Cancer. 2007;109:536–41.

Umekita Y, Hiipakka RA, Kokontis JM, Liao S. Human prostate tumor growth in athymic mice: inhibition by androgens and stimulation by finasteride. Proc Natl Acad Sci USA. 1996;93:11802–7.

Wang C, Nieschlag E, Swerdloff R, et al. Investigation, treatment, and monitoring of late-onset hypogonadism in males: ISA, ISSAM, EAU, EAA, and ASA recommendations. Eur Urol. 2009;55:121–30.

Chapter 8
The Role of Testosterone in the Metabolic Syndrome in Men

Farid Saad

Introduction

The metabolic syndrome is a cluster of components which have been identified from many epidemiological studies as the most important risk factors for cardiovascular diseases and type 2 diabetes. Different definitions have slightly different cut-off levels, but all contain the same components:

- Abdominal obesity
- Dyslipidemia, i.e., elevated triglycerides and decreased HDL cholesterol
- High blood pressure
- Insulin resistance

These risk factors are also called "the silent killers" because they can be present for many years without any obvious symptoms. Nobody can "feel" high triglycerides or low HDL, nobody notices when the blood sugar exceeds a certain threshold, and even high blood pressure can go unnoticed for a long time. These symptoms can only be detected and diagnosed upon measurement of laboratory values or – in case of hypertension – by measuring blood pressure. Abdominal obesity is, of course, visible, but it is certainly not understood as what it really is – a most serious risk factor for cardiovascular health. If left undiagnosed and untreated, the metabolic syndrome leads progressively to the manifestation of cardiovascular diseases and type 2 diabetes.

F. Saad, DVM, Ph.D.
Department of Endocrinology, Gulf Medical University & Bayer Pharma Germany, Ajman, UAE

Hang Tuah Medical University, Surabaya, Indonesia

Men's Healthcare Scientific Affairs c/o Bayer Schering Pharma AG, Berlin D-13342, Germany
e-mail: farid.saad@bayer.com

P.H.C. Lim (ed.), *Men's Health*,
DOI 10.1007/978-1-4471-4766-4_8, © Springer-Verlag London 2013

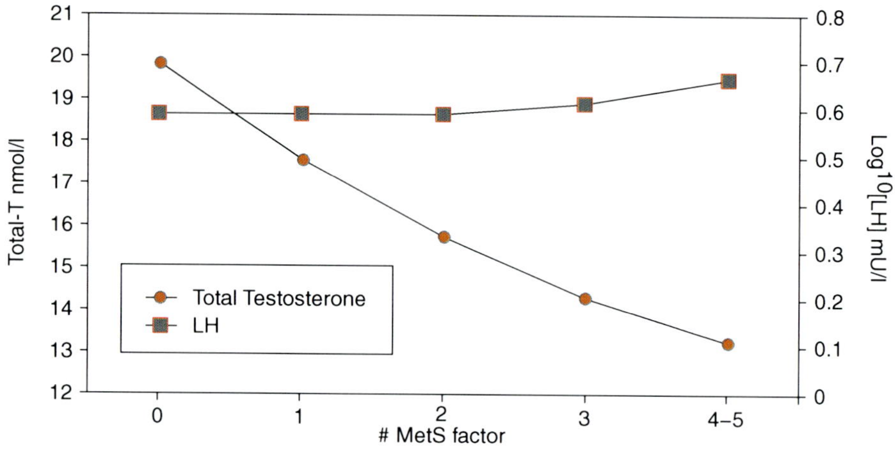

Fig. 8.1 Total testosterone (*T*) and LH (log. transformed) levels as a function of metabolic syndrome (*MetS*) factors in a consecutive series of 1,535 patients presenting for sexual dysfunction (Corona et al. 2008)

Epidemiology

Epidemiological studies – both cross-sectional and longitudinal – have shown associations between plasma levels of testosterone and the metabolic syndrome. Men with the metabolic syndrome have lower testosterone than men without the metabolic syndrome. This holds true not only for the metabolic syndrome as a whole but also for every component of the metabolic syndrome. However, the more components of the metabolic syndrome a man has, the lower his testosterone (Fig. 8.1).

Moreover, it has been demonstrated in longitudinal studies that men who at baseline have low testosterone but no metabolic syndrome have a higher probability to develop the metabolic syndrome than men with normal testosterone. Vice versa, men who have the metabolic syndrome but normal testosterone are more likely to have testosterone deficiency later on. Therefore, low testosterone is a predictor for the metabolic syndrome, and the metabolic syndrome is a predictor for low testosterone.

A very unique opportunity to study the effects of testosterone on the metabolic syndrome is provided by the standard treatment for advanced prostate cancer: These patients undergo surgical or medical castration, i.e., their testosterone is suppressed to severely hypogonadal levels. These men develop within a very short period of time – a matter of weeks – all the symptoms which are summarized in the metabolic syndrome: increase in fat mass (and simultaneous decrease in muscle mass), increase of total cholesterol and triglycerides, increase in blood pressure, and – most dramatically – onset or an increase in insulin resistance. It is now very clear that men on androgen deprivation therapy (ADT) have a significantly increased risk of cardiovascular diseases and type 2 diabetes (Figs. 8.2 and 8.3).

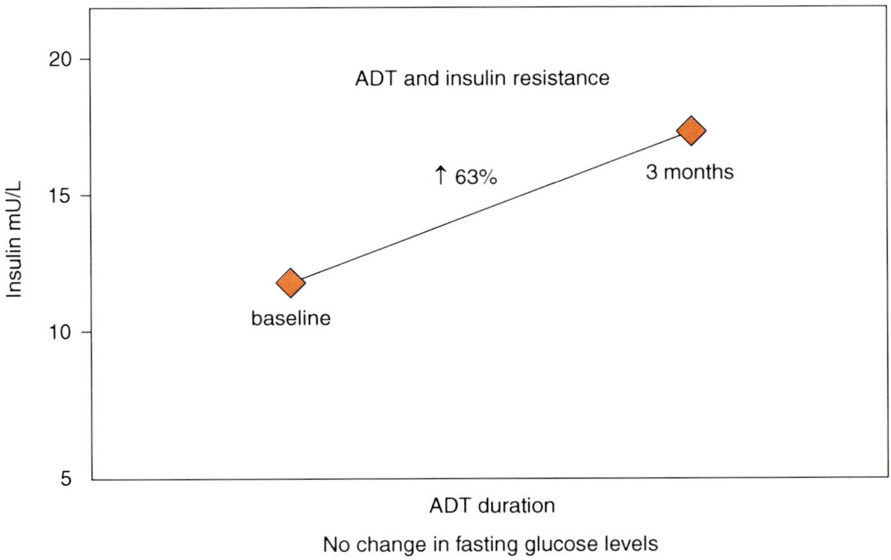

Fig. 8.2 Hyperinsulinemia developing within 3 months of androgen deprivation therapy (*ADT*) (Basaria 2008)

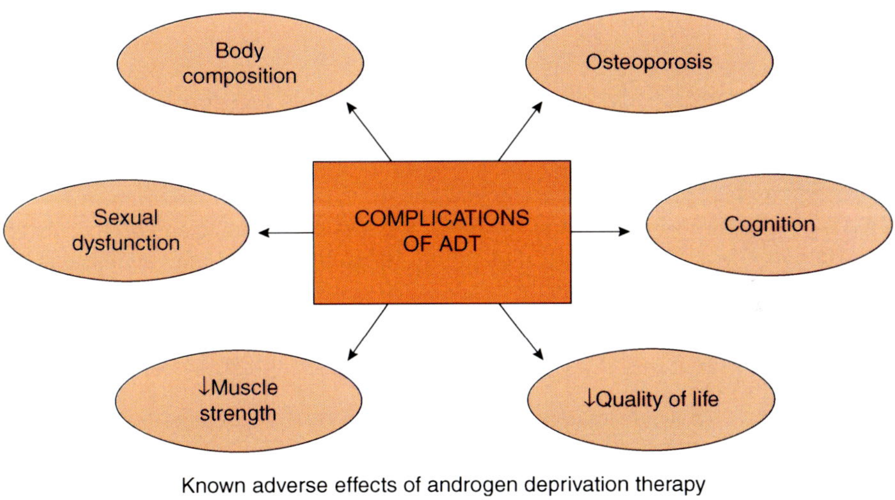

Fig. 8.3 Androgen deprivation therapy adverse effects (Basaria 2008)

Role of Testosterone

When men with the metabolic syndrome and testosterone deficiency receive testosterone treatment, every single factor of the metabolic syndrome improves.

Men experience changes in their body composition. Upon normalization of testosterone levels, fat mass decreases, in particular the abdominal fat which can be

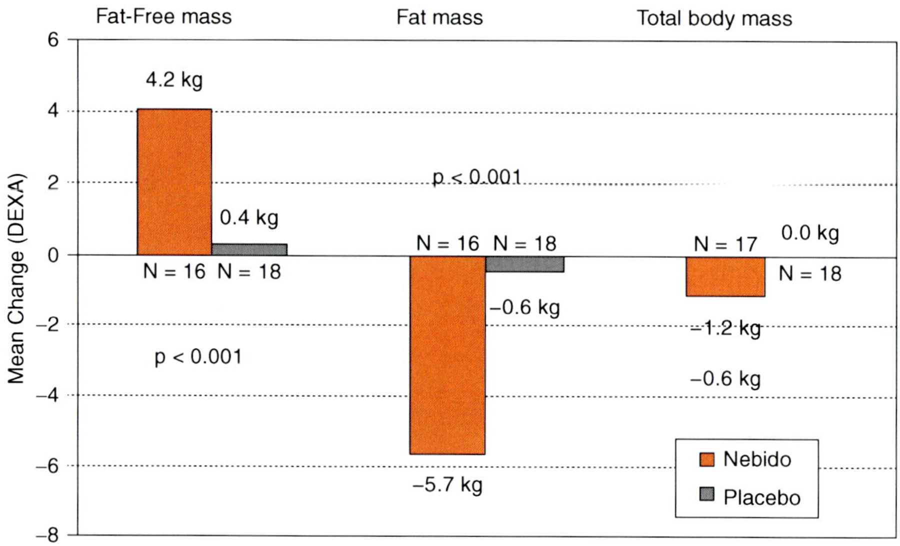

Fig. 8.4 Testosterone therapy with Nebido® improved body composition in elderly men (Svartberg et al. 2008)

easily measured by taking the waist circumference. Testosterone seems to selectively have a better effect on abdominal (or visceral) fat compared to subcutaneous fat although subcutaneous fat also responds to testosterone (Fig. 8.4). In a study where men received 1 year of treatment with long-acting testosterone injections, they lost an amazing 5.7 kg of fat mass. At the same time, their muscle mass increased by 4.2 kg. The increase in muscle mass is of equal importance as the muscle is the organ where most of the blood sugar is metabolized and more muscle translates into better glucose metabolization. In another study, after 15 months of treatment with testosterone, men lost 8 cm waist circumference, and a third study showed that, when testosterone treatment was combined with better diet and exercise, the reduction of waist circumference after 1 year reached an astonishing 14.6 cm (Fig. 8.5).

When metabolic syndrome patients are treated with testosterone, their lipid pattern improves. Total cholesterol and LDL cholesterol and triglycerides are reduced (Fig. 8.6), whereas HDL cholesterol increases. This may be a result of the changes in body composition.

In the early 1990s, for the first time a reduction of diastolic blood pressure upon testosterone treatment was reported. More than 10 years later, several studies could confirm these results, and reductions in both systolic and diastolic blood pressure were repeatedly demonstrated in men receiving testosterone therapy. The magnitude of the decrease is clinically meaningful and can reach approximately 10 mmHg both in systolic and diastolic blood pressure (Fig. 8.7). Several mechanisms can be involved in this effect of testosterone. The improvement of Blood Pressure is due to

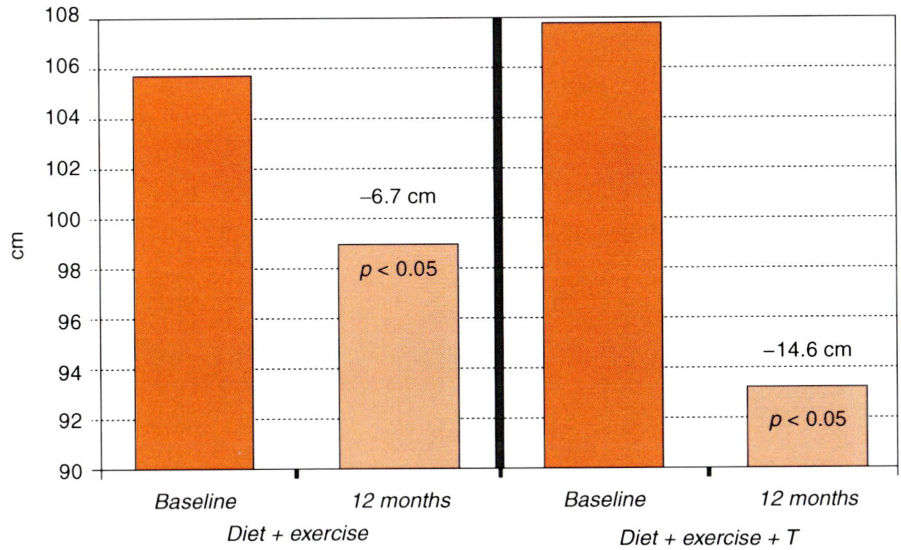

Fig. 8.5 Waist circumference in 32 hypogonadal men with newly diagnosed type 2 diabetes (Heufelder et al. 2009)

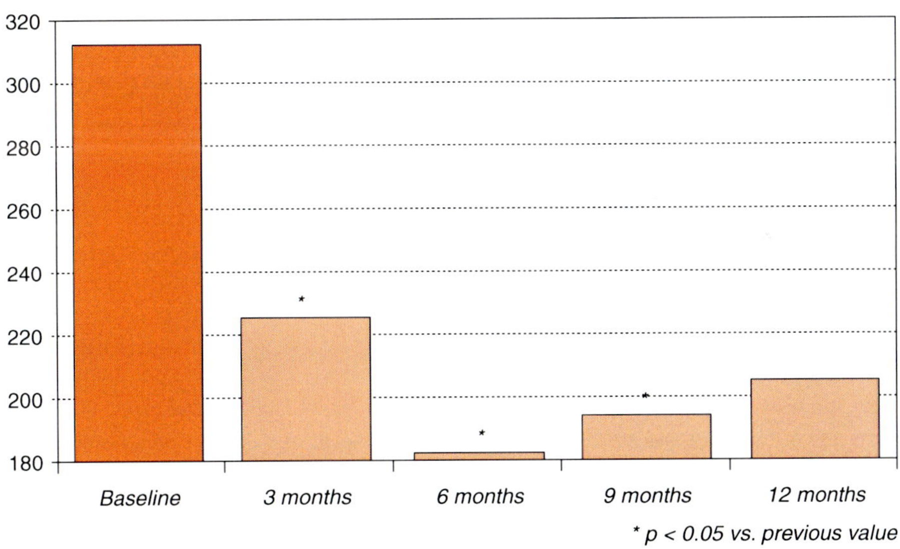

Fig. 8.6 Triglycerides (mg/dl) (Normal: <180 mg/dl) in 28 hypogonadal ED patients (median age: 64 years, range: 54–76) treated with TU (Nebido) for 12 months (Saad et al. 2007)

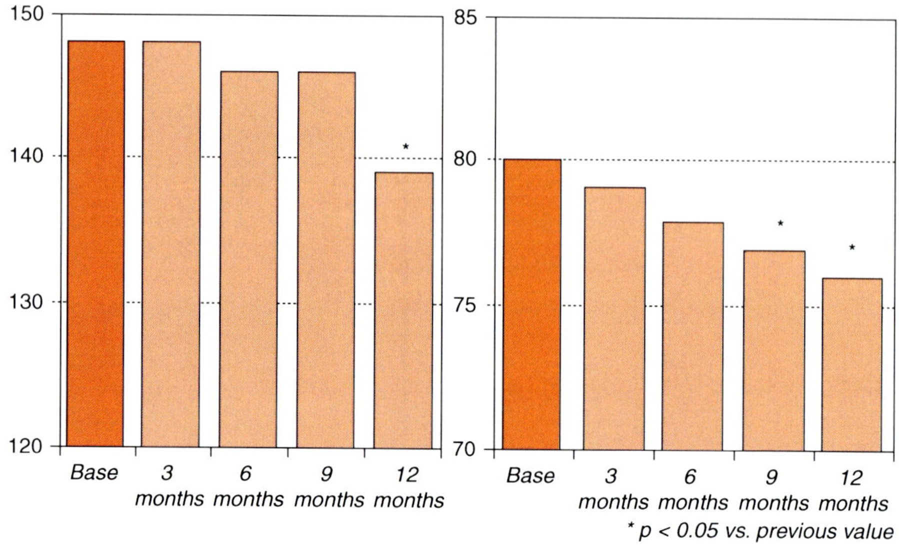

Fig. 8.7 Systolic and diastolic blood pressure (mmHg) in 28 hypogonadal ED patients (median age: 64 years, range: 54–76) treated with TU (Nebido) or 12 months (Saad et al. 2007)

the properties of testosterone as a vasodilator the properties of testosterone as a vasodilator: by increase of endothelial nitric oxide production and by decrease of endothelin-1, testosterone acts as a vasodilator. Finally, testosterone has anticoagulatory effects by reducing fibrinogen and plasminogen activator inhibitor-1 (PAI-1).

Testosterone improves insulin sensitivity. In an elegant experimental study, healthy men received a GnRH antagonist which leads to immediate suppression of testosterone to castration levels. Then these men received either GnRH or HCG to stimulate their own endogenous testosterone production. Insulin sensitivity was measured by the gold standard method, the hyperinsulinemic-euglycemic clamp technique. The higher their testosterone rose, the better their insulin sensitivity became. This occurred within 48 h, a period too short for any changes in body composition. One could conclude from this study that testosterone has a direct, dose-dependent effect on insulin sensitivity.

Numerous other studies in men with metabolic syndrome as well as type 2 diabetes have shown that testosterone reduces glucose, insulin, and HbA_{1c}. In combination with diet and exercise, testosterone reduced HbA_{1c} by 1.2 % without any other antidiabetic medication.

Testosterone plays a central role in the metabolic syndrome. The fact that testosterone improves every single component of the metabolic syndrome supports a causative role of this hormone in the pathophysiology of the metabolic syndrome. Once the results from larger ongoing studies become available, testosterone can be a powerful tool in the treatment of the metabolic syndrome and, particularly, obesity in men.

References

Basaria S. Androgen deprivation therapy, insulin resistance, and cardiovascular mortality: an inconvenient truth. J Androl. 2008;29(5):534–9.

Corona G, Forti G, Maggi M. Why can patients with erectile dysfunction be considered lucky? The association with testosterone deficiency and metabolic syndrome. Aging Male. 2008;11: 193–9.

Haider A, Gooren L, Padungtod P, Saad F. Concurrent improvement of the metabolic syndrome and lower urinary tract symptoms upon normalisation of plasma testosterone levels in hypogonadal elderly men. Andrologia. 2009;41:7–13.

Heufelder A, Saad F, Bunck M, Gooren L. 52-week treatment with diet and exercise plus transdermal testosterone reverses the metabolic syndrome and improves glycaemic control in men with newly diagnosed type 2 diabetes and subnormal plasma testosterone. J Androl. 2009;30:726–63. Epub 2009 Jul 3.

Pitteloud N, Hardin M, Dwyer A, Valassi E, Yialamas M, Elahi D, Hayes F. Increasing insulin resistance is associated with a decrease in Leydig cell testosterone secretion in men. J Clin Endocrinol Metab. 2005;90:2636–41.

Saad F, Gooren L. The role of testosterone in the metabolic syndrome: a review. J Steroid Biochem Mol Biol. 2009;114:40–3.

Saad F, Gooren L, Haider A, Yassin A. An exploratory study of the effects of 12 month administration of the novel long-acting testosterone undecanoate on measures of sexual function and the metabolic syndrome. Arch Androl J Reprod Syst. 2007;53:353–7.

Svartberg J, et al. Int J Import Res. 2008;20:378–87.

Traish AM, Guay A, Feeley R, Saad F. The dark side of testosterone deficiency: I. Metabolic syndrome and erectile dysfunction. J Androl. 2009;30:10–22.

Chapter 9
The Testosterone and ED (or Sexual Function) Connection

Farid Saad

Introduction

The role of testosterone in male sexual function has been controversially discussed in the literature. The control of libido by testosterone is a well-established knowledge (Fig. 9.1). Assessment of libido in hypogonadal men treated with testosterone invariably results in an increase. Recent data have shown that sexual thoughts and fantasy are restored within as little as 3 weeks in men receiving testosterone treatment (Fig. 9.2). Also for a long time, testosterone has been known to be closely associated with the number and quality of nocturnal erections. The decrease of morning erections is one of the key symptoms of hypogonadism (Fig. 9.3). However, testosterone was not considered to be a successful treatment for erectile dysfunction (ED) with the exception of a very small group of patients with extremely low testosterone levels as an actual cause for ED. This opinion was even enhanced by the introduction of PDE5 inhibitors which made testosterone therapy for ED almost forgotten (Wespes et al. 2006).

Animal Experiments (Traish and Guay 2006)

Animal experiments have shown that castration causes changes in the penis, i.e., a reduction in smooth muscle content and an increase in connective tissue. This could be restored by testosterone replenishment. After castration, an accumulation of fat cells was observed in the space between corpus cavernosum smooth muscle and tunica albuginea. These fat cells which impair the veno-occlusive

F. Saad, DVM, Ph.D.
Department of Endocrinology, Gulf Medical University & Bayer Pharma Germany, Ajman, UAE

Hang Tuah Medical University, Surabaya, Indonesia

Men's Healthcare Scientific Affairs c/o Bayer
Schering Pharma AG, Berlin D-13342, Germany
e-mail: farid.saad@bayer.com

P.H.C. Lim (ed.), *Men's Health*,
DOI 10.1007/978-1-4471-4766-4_9,

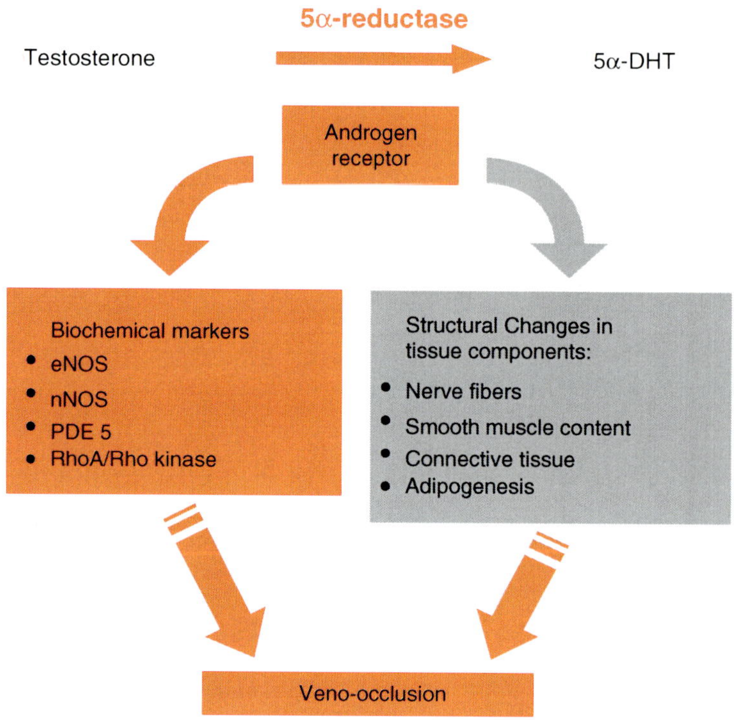

Fig. 9.1 Testosterone and veno-occlusion in cavernosal tissue

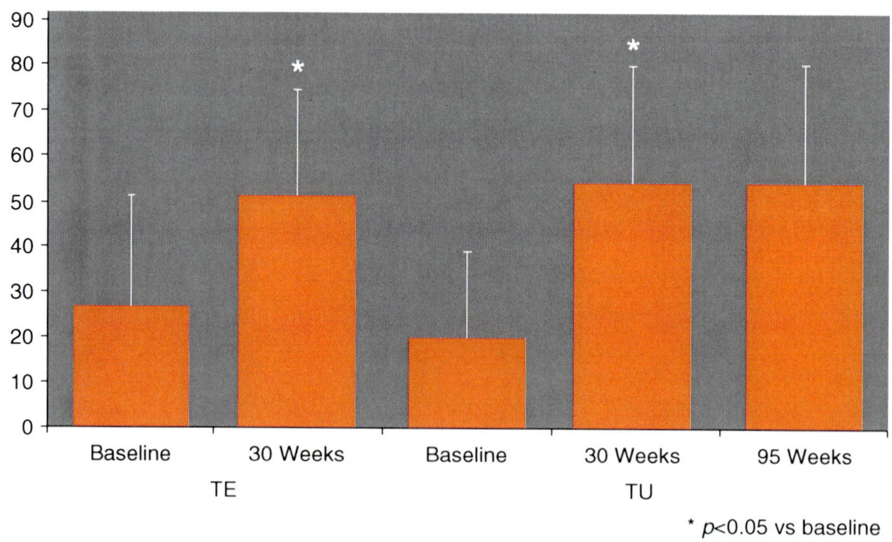

Fig. 9.2 Sexual interest and desire on a visual analog scale before and after treatment with TE and TU (Nebido®) in 40 hypogonadal men (Jockenhoevel et al. 2009)

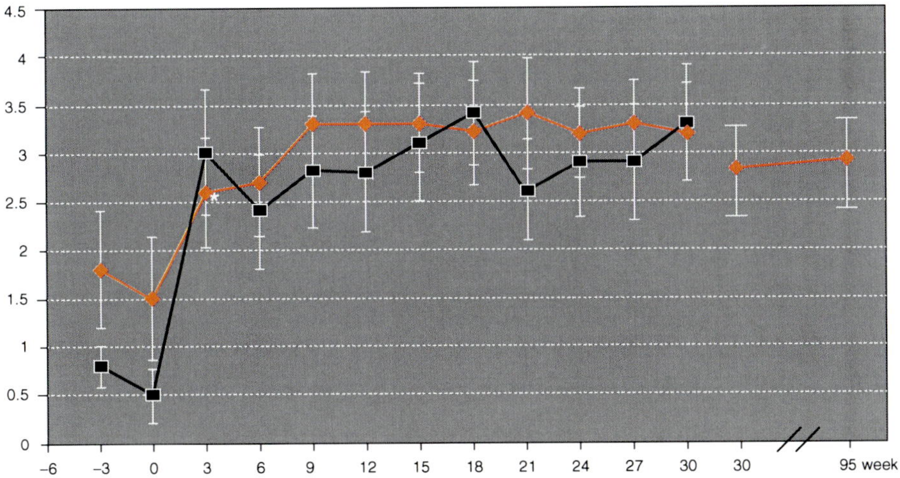

Fig. 9.3 Spontaneous morning erectionsper week after repeated injections of TE or TU in 40 hypogonadal men (mean age 41, range: 18–74 years) (Rajfer et al. 1988)

mechanism – the "trapping" of the blood within the penis when erection occurs – disappeared after testosterone treatment. An interesting study in the rabbit model contributed further to elucidate the role of testosterone in erection. Testosterone-deficient animals showed a diminished erectile response to electrical pelvic nerve stimulation. When these rabbits received the PDE5 inhibitor vardenafil, they showed markedly reduced response. The histological analysis of the corpus cavernosum smooth muscle revealed a shift in the ratio from smooth muscle to connective tissue. This indicates a loss of functionality and elasticity impairing the veno-occlusive mechanism. Another rat study performed in China showed a structural change of the tunica albuginea in castrated animals which would also contribute to a functional loss of the veno-occlusive mechanism. Finally, the structure of the cavernosal nerve deteriorates after castration, which can be reversed by testosterone in the animal model (Traish et al. 2009).

Apart from penile structure, testosterone was also found to have an impact on biochemical functional parameters. It not only influences nitric oxide synthesis and release but also the expression of the enzyme phosphodiesterase type 5 which is the substrate for PDE5 inhibitors. Thereby, testosterone has a role in facilitating the effect of PDE5 inhibitors.

Smooth Muscle and Veno-occlusive Dysfunction
(Yassin et al. 2006)

Simultaneously with the experimental results, clinical results were published confirming the findings in animal research. Interestingly, investigators from Turkey showed that men with erectile dysfunction (ED) had a reduced content of smooth

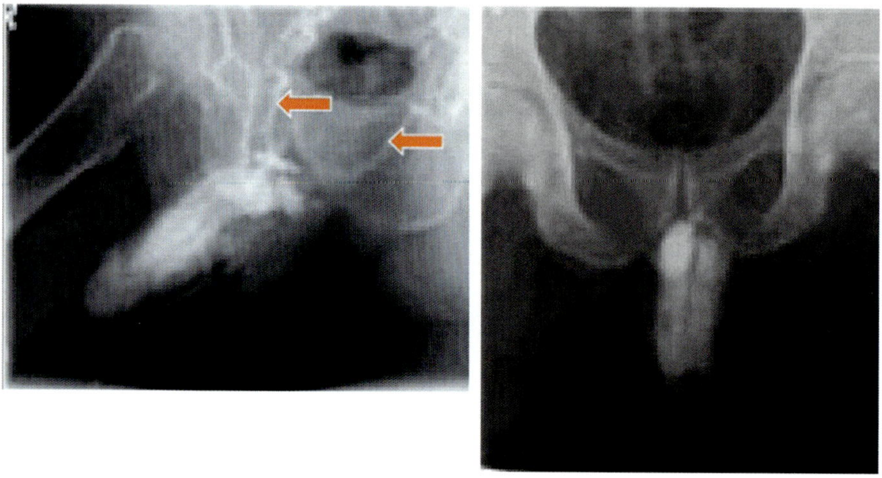

Fig. 9.4 Cavernosography in a 56-year-old hypogonadal man ($T = 1.8$ ng/mL, 6.2 nmol/L) with type 2 diabetes, metabolic syndrome and erectile dysfunction at baseline and after 12 weeks of testosterone therapy with i.m. testosterone undecanoate (Nebido®) (*arrows*) shows point of leakage (Yassin and Saad 2006)

muscle cells, endothelial cells, and elastic fibers in their penile corpus cavernosum compared to men with intact erectile function. And again, they also demonstrated that men on castration therapy for advanced prostate cancer had a reduction of penile length correlating with the duration of testosterone withdrawal. This suggests that anatomical changes occur in men equally as in experimental animals. Finally, one of the most severe forms of ED caused by venous leakage was treated tentatively in two independent pilot studies in Germany and Russia. Patients with venous leak are considered candidates for penile implants, an irreversible ultima ratio treatment. Both investigators could "repair" venous leak in approximately 50 % of their patients by restoring testosterone levels back to normal, suggesting that the impaired veno-occlusive mechanism could be reversed, very likely a cause of restoring the structure of corpus cavernosum and tunica albuginea (Fig. 9.4) (Kurbatov et al. 2008).

PDE5 Inhibitors

Testosterone was routinely measured in diabetic ED patients in Russia (Fig. 9.5). The authors found a highly significant difference between PDE5 inhibitor responders and nonresponders. Nonresponders, without exception, had testosterone levels in the hypogonadal range, whereas the responders were in the normal range. When they treated these nonresponders additionally with testosterone, they saw clear improvement in scores of the International Index of Erectile Function (IIEF). These scores improved under testosterone supplementation and went back to baseline after

	PDE-5 i non-responders $n = 120$	PDE-5 i responders $n = 100$	PDE-5 i $n = 120$ $n = 100$
	Mean ± SD	Mean ± SD	p value
Total testosterone (nmol/L)	6.9 ± 1.3 (4.5 – 9.6)	18.6 ± 1.2 (14.3 – 29.1)	<0.001

Fig. 9.5 Different testosterone levels in diabetic responders and non-responders to PDE-5 inhibitors (Kalinchenko et al. 2003)

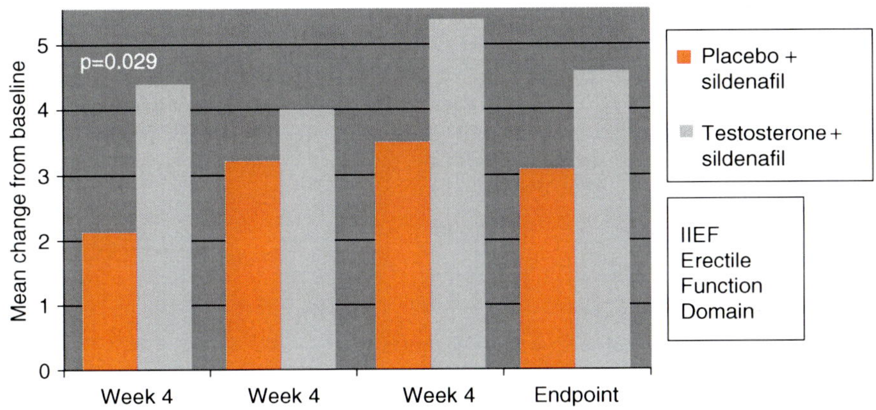

Fig. 9.6 Twelve week testosterone therapy (Testogel®) converts sildenafil 100 mg non-responders to responders in men with hypogonadism (tT <14 nmol/L) and erectile dysfunction

cessation of testosterone treatment. These results were confirmed in a multicenter, double-blind, placebo-controlled trial in the USA. PDE5 inhibitor nonresponders received 3 months treatment with testosterone. Patients had initial testosterone levels <400 ng/dL (approximately 14 nmol/L) which is considered within the low normal range (Fig. 9.6). The erectile function domain of the IIEF improved significantly after as little as 4 weeks and was maintained on this high level over the full 3 months. These findings were confirmed by an Italian study in which additionally penile blood flow was measured with analogous results.

Yassin et al. in Germany went "the other way." In accordance with EAU guidelines, in all men presenting with ED, testosterone levels were measured before treatment. Hypogonadal men received testosterone treatment. After 3 months of treatment with testosterone undecanoate injections alone, 54 % of the patients regained their erectile function. Sexual desire improved in all patients independent of their improvement of erections. After 8 months of treatment, this proportion increased only by another 4 % to a total of 58 %, suggesting that an optimal treatment effect with testosterone alone can be expected after 3 months. Then, a PDE5 inhibitor should be added to relieve the remaining patients of their symptoms (Fig. 9.7).

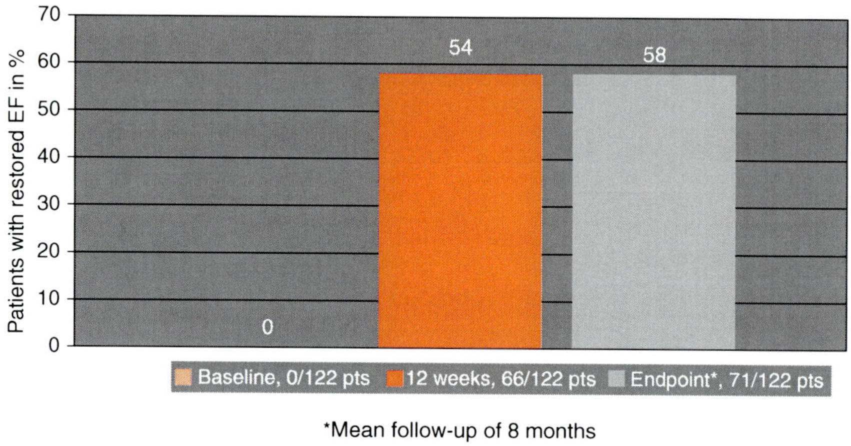

Fig. 9.7 Patients with normal erectile function in % at baseline, after 12 weeks and at endpoint* of therapy with Nebido® (122 hypogonadal ED patients) (Yassin and Saad 2006)

This approach was chosen in another study in Israel, when hypogonadal men with ED received testosterone treatment first. About two thirds responded with normalization of erectile function. The remaining men were then treated with PDE5 inhibitors and responded successfully to the combination treatment.

New Perspective

All components of the metabolic syndrome are risk factors for erectile dysfunction, and ED may not only be an early warning marker for cardiometabolic diseases but also the most important bothersome symptom that drives men to the doctor's office (Corona et al. 2008). ED, testosterone deficiency, and metabolic syndrome are intertwined, and ED may be the reason to detect cardiovascular risk factors which were previously unknown. Today, ED is seen as a symptom rather than a disease, and ED should prompt physicians to look for underlying conditions which may save the patient's life. Measuring testosterone is one of the recommended steps to assess the patient presenting with ED.

Conclusion

In summary, structural and functional changes in the penis may be caused by low testosterone levels and can – at least partly – be restored by testosterone treatment. Other significant impact on psychosexual parameters can be expected. Testosterone seems to facilitate the effect of PDE5 inhibitors by restoring the smooth muscle compartment. It could be considered as an additional treatment for patients in whom these compounds have failed.

References

Corona G, Forti G, Maggi M. Why can patients with erectile dysfunction be considered lucky? The association with testosterone deficiency and metabolic syndrome. Aging Male. 2008;11:193–9.

Jockenhoevel F, Minnemann T, Schubert M, Freude S, Huebler D, Schumann C, Christoph A, Ernst M, Gooren L. Time table of effects of testosterone administration to hypogonadal men on variables of sex and mood. Aging Male. 2009;12:113–8.

Kalinchenko SY, Kozlov G, Gontcharov N, Katsiya G. Oral testosterone undecanoate reverses erectile dysfunction associated with diabetes mellitus in patients failing on sildenafil citrate therapy alone. Aging Male. 2003;6:94–9.

Kurbatov D, Kuznetsky J, Traish A. Testosterone improves erectile function in hypogonadal patients with venous leakage. J Androl. 2008;29:630–7.

Rajfer J, Rosciszewski A, Mehringer M. Prevalence of corporeal venous leakage in impotent men. J Urol. 1988;140:69–71.

Traish AM, Guay AT. Are androgens critical for penile erection in humans? Examining the clinical and preclinical evidence. J Sex Med. 2006;3:382–407.

Traish AM, Guay A, Feeley R, Saad F. The dark side of testosterone deficiency: I. Metabolic syndrome and erectile dysfunction. J Androl. 2009;30:10–22.

Wespes E, Amar E, Hatzichristou D, Hatzimouratidis K, Montorsi M, Pryor J, Vardi Y. EAU guidelines on erectile dysfunction: an update. Eur Urol. 2006;49:806–15.

Yassin AA, Saad F. Treatment of sexual dysfunction of hypogonadal patients with long-acting testosterone undecanoate (Nebido®). World J Urol. 2006;24:639–44.

Yassin AA, Traish A, Saad F. Testosterone undecanoate restores erectile function in a subset of patients with venous leakage: a series of case reports. J Sex Med. 2006;3:727–35.

Chapter 10
Treating Hypogonadism Associated with Erectile Dysfunction

Ng Kok Kit

The Massachusetts Male Aging Study (Gray et al. 1991) found that 52 % of men older than 40 years old had some degree of erectile failure. The same study also confirmed that free testosterone decreases 1.2 % per year and bioavailable testosterone decreases 1.0 % per year and SHBG increases 1.2 % per year between the ages of 40 and 70. Both erectile dysfunction and hypogonadism increase in incidence with age. Erectile dysfunction has several possible etiologies, including vasculogenic, neurogenic, psychogenic, or endocrine cause. A major component of endocrine cause is late-onset hypogonadism.

The European Association of Urology guidelines for erectile dysfunction suggested that testosterone level, including calculated free and bioavailable testosterone level, should be measured as part of the basic laboratory workup for erectile dysfunction. The question is how should a patient with late-onset hypogonadism and erectile dysfunction be treated?

Role of Testosterone in Erection

Testosterone has several roles in the process of erection (Mikhail 2006). It has a role at the central level as well as at the end organ level.

Erections are dependent on central nervous system-mediated actions, such as the excitability associated with central erectile signaling, synaptic interconnections, and the peripheral neurotransmitter pool, which are all mediated by physiologic testosterone homeostasis.

Ng.K. Kit, MBBS (Singapore), FRCS (Glas), FRCS (Edin), FAMS (Urology)
Department of Urology, Changi General Hospital, Singapore, Singapore

Andropause and Men's Health Clinic, Changi General Hospital, Singapore, Singapore
e-mail: kok_kit_ng@cgh.com.sg

P.H.C. Lim (ed.), *Men's Health*,
DOI 10.1007/978-1-4471-4766-4_10,

At the level of the end organ, testosterone acts at two areas – in the nitric oxide pathway, allowing for cGMP formation, through positive modulation of nitric oxide synthase, and through the regulation of PDE5 expression.

ED with Low Testosterone Levels

Since testosterone acts at the central and the end organ level in erectile physiology, the lack of testosterone causes erectile dysfunction at these two levels.

In the brain, low testosterone level is associated with a reduction in erectile signaling. Testosterone replacement in hypogonadal patients has resulted in a significant increase in brain activity in response to sexual stimulation to levels similar to those seen in men with normal testosterone (Park et al. 2001).

At the end organ level, it was found that following castration in rats, testosterone replacement was able to reverse the atrophy of cavernosal nerves (Rogers et al. 2003) and to restore the release of the vasodilator nitric oxide in response to cavernosal nerve stimulation, as well as the content of both endothelial and neuronal nitric oxide synthase in cavernosal tissue (Martin et al. 1999). Testosterone replacement is also able to normalize active RhoA/Rho kinase signaling pathways (Vignozzi et al. 2007) in cavernosal tissues after castration. Moreover, normal testosterone levels prevent cavernous smooth muscle apoptosis. In castrated animals, it has been found that there is an accumulation of adipocytes (Traish et al. 2005) in the subtunical region of the corpus cavernosum.

Testosterone deficiency also affects the PDE5 expression at the end organ level. Castration of rats significantly reduces PDE5 gene and protein expression in the corpus cavernosum (Zhang et al. 2005), as well as the erectile response to electrostimulation.

Testosterone Monotherapy for ED

Studies on testosterone monotherapy for the treatment of ED have generally yielded positive results (Jain et al. 2000), although there are many limitations in such studies. Studies (Zitzmann et al. 2002) have also shown that testosterone supplementation is an effective treatment for hypogonadal ED and may provide increased vascular reactivity. On the other hand, erections are still possible in hypogonadal conditions (Morelli et al. 2005) in which a decreased cGMP formation, because of impaired nitric oxide production, is counterbalanced by a reduced cGMP hydrolysis.

A meta-analysis of the effects of testosterone on sexual function (Isidori et al. 2005) has been carried out by Isidori et al. Testosterone supplementation moderately improved the number of nocturnal erections, sexual thoughts, motivation, number of successful intercourses, scores of erectile function, and overall satisfaction compared with placebo. Testosterone did not have any effect on erectile function in eugonadal men.

Combination of Testosterone and PDE5 Inhibitors for ED

Phosphodiesterase type V inhibitors (PDE5 inhibitors) are drugs like sildenafil (Viagra), vardenafil (Levitra), and tadalafil (Cialis) that have revolutionized the treatment of erectile dysfunction. They act by inhibiting PDE5, which breaks down cGMP. This in turn results in an increase of nitric oxide, which is an important mediator in erection. Clinical studies have shown the efficacy and safety of all these drugs that have made them the first line and mainstay of therapy of men with erectile dysfunction.

However, 23–50 % of patients do not respond to PDE5 inhibitors (Salonia et al. 2003) alone. Testosterone, through both its central and end organ effects on erection, has been studied when used in combination with PDE5 inhibitors. Different studies (Shabsigh et al. 2004) have shown that testosterone therapy is able to improve erectile function and the response to PDE5 inhibitors in patients with ED and hypogonadism. It has also been shown in some studies (Aversa et al. 2003) that testosterone supplementation also increased the International Index of Erectile Function (IIEF) scores even in eugonadal patients who did not respond to sildenafil alone, by improving sexual desire and orgasmic function and by increasing arterial inflow to the penis during sexual stimulation. Other studies have also confirmed the beneficial effects of combination therapy in patients with comorbid conditions. Administration of intramuscular testosterone and oral sildenafil in end-stage renal failure patients (Chatterjee et al. 2004) who had renal transplants or renal dialysis was found to be efficacious. Oral testosterone has been reported to reverse ED associated with type II diabetes (Kalinchenko et al. 2003) in patients failing sildenafil therapy alone.

In conclusion, testosterone and PDE5 inhibitor combination therapy improves the response to PDE5 inhibitors (Greco et al. 2006) in patients previously not responding to PDE5 inhibitor therapy alone and in whom testosterone levels at baseline are in the hypogonadal or normal–low adult range (i.e., late-onset hypogonadism).

What Should I Do?

Initial Assessment

Patients can present first with suspicion of late-onset hypogonadism or come in with ED.

When they come in for screening for late-onset hypogonadism, they usually have some symptoms suggestive of "andropause." A major component of andropause is actually sexual symptoms, whether it is erectile dysfunction or decreased libido. If the patient complains of sexual symptom, a good way of quantifying his symptoms would be through the International Index of Erectile Function (IIEF). It is much more convenient to use the abbreviated form called *IIEF-5* (see Fig. 10.1), which consists only of five items in the questionnaire. That way, patients can be classified into mild, moderate, or severe erectile dysfunction.

These questions assess your erectile and sexual function.

Over the past 6 months:

1. How do you rate your confidence that you could get and keep an erection		Very low 1 ☐	Low 2 ☐	Moderate 3 ☐	High 4 ☐	Very high 5 ☐
2. When you had erections with sexual stimulation, how often were your erections hard enough for penetration?	No sexual activity 0 ☐	Almost never / never 1 ☐	A few times (much less than half the time) 2 ☐	Sometimes (about half the time) 3 ☐	Most times (much more than half the time) 4 ☐	Almost always / always 5 ☐
3. During sexual intercourse, how often were you able to maintain your erection after you had penetrated (entered) your partner?	Did not attempt intercourse 0 ☐	Almost never / never 1 ☐	A few times (much less than half the time) 2 ☐	Sometimes (about half the time) 3 ☐	Most times (much more than half the time) 4 ☐	Almost always / always 5 ☐
4. During sexual intercourse, how difficult was it to maintain your erection to completion of intercourse?	Did not attempt intercourse 0 ☐	Extremel y difficult 1 ☐	Very difficult 2 ☐	Difficult 3 ☐	Slightly difficult 4 ☐	Not difficult 5 ☐
5. When you attempted sexual intercourse, how often was it satisfactory for you?	Did not attempt intercourse 0 ☐	Almost never / never 1 ☐	A few times (much less than half the time) 2 ☐	Sometimes (about half the time) 3 ☐	Most times (much more than half the time) 4 ☐	Almost always / always 5 ☐

Total score: No ED (22-25); mild ED (17-21); mild to moderate ED (12-16); moderate ED (8-11); severeED (5-7)

Fig. 10.1 International index of erectile function (IIEF)

When the patient presents with ED, a history should be taken to look for other signs of andropause. A telltale sign would be decrease in libido. EAU guidelines recommend a baseline hormone profile. This includes *testosterone* level, together with *SHBG* and *albumin* levels if free and bioavailable testosterone are to be calculated. Serum *prolactin* is also performed to look for pituitary disorders. Gonadotrophins – follicle-stimulating hormone (FSH) and luteinizing hormone (LH) – can also be measured but are optional.

If the patient presents with ED as his main complaint, PDE5 inhibitors can be started first to look for a therapeutic response.

If the patient also has a low testosterone level, testosterone therapy can be initiated at the same time or at a later period after a complete discussion is performed with the patient. It should be noted that unlike PDE5 inhibitor therapy which would show an almost immediate improvement to erectile function, the patient will need to wait for at least 6 weeks to see any improvement from testosterone therapy.

At Follow-Up

What happens during follow-up after the patient has been diagnosed to have late-onset hypogonadism and put on therapy?

If the patient is on PDE5 monotherapy and his erection is still poor, his PDE5 therapy can be combined with testosterone therapy.

Vice versa, if he is on testosterone therapy alone and his major concern is still his poor erection, PDE5 inhibitor therapy can be started.

Some hypogonadal patients who have been on combination therapy later find that they do not need to depend on PDE5 inhibitor to help with their erection.

If a patient is on combination PDE5 inhibitor and testosterone therapy and finds that his erection is still poor and ED being his predominant concern, he may need second-line treatment of his ED. Second-line treatment would include modalities like vacuum device therapy or intracavernosal injection. When second-line treatments fail, he can opt for a penile implant.

References

Aversa A, Isidori AM, Spera G, Lenzi A, Fabbri A. Androgens improve cavernous vasodilation and response to sildenafil in patient with erectile dysfunction. Clin Endocrinol. 2003;58:632–8.

Chatterjee R, Wood S, McGarrigle HH, Lees WR, Ralph DJ, Neild GH. A novel therapy with testosterone and sildenafil for erectile dysfunction in patients on renal dialysis or after renal transplantation. J Fam Plann Reprod Health Care. 2004;30:88–90.

Gray A, Feldman HA, McKinlay JB, et al. Age, disease and changing sex hormone levels in middle-aged men: results of the Massachusetts Male Aging Study. J Clin Endocrinol Metab. 1991;73:1016–25.

Greco EA, Spera G, Aversa A. Combining testosterone and PDE5 inhibitors in erectile dysfunction: basic rationale and clinical evidences. Eur Urol. 2006;50:940–7.

Isidori AM, Giannetta E, Gianfrilli D, et al. Effects of testosterone on sexual function in men: results of a meta-analysis. Clin Endocrinol. 2005;63:381–94.

Jain P, Rademaker AW, McVary KT. Testosterone supplementation for erectile dysfunction: results of a metaanalysis. J Urol. 2000;164:371–5.

Kalinchenko SY, Kozlov GI, Gontcharov NP, Katsiya GV. Oral testosterone undecanoate reverses erectile dysfunction associated with diabetes mellitus in patients failing on sildenafil citrate therapy alone. Aging Male. 2003;6:94–9.

Martin R, Escrig A, Abreu P, Mas M. Androgen-dependent nitric oxide release in rat penis correlates with levels of constitutive nitric oxide synthase isoenzymes. Biol Reprod. 1999;61:1012–6.

Mikhail N. Does testosterone have a role to play in erectile function? Am J Med. 2006;119:373–82.

Morelli A, Filippi S, Zhang XH, et al. Peripheral regulatory mechanisms in erection. Int J Androl. 2005;28:23–7.

Park K, Seo JJ, Kang HK, Ryu SB, Kim HJ, Jeong GW. A new potential of blood oxygenation level dependent (BOLD) functional MRI for evaluating cerebral centers of penile erection. Int J Impot Res. 2001;13:73–81.

Rogers RS, Graziottin TM, Lin C-S, Kan YW, Lue TF. Intracavernosal vascular endothelial growth factor (VEGF) injection and adeno-associated virus-mediated VEGF gene therapy prevent and reverse venogenic erectile dysfunction in rats. Int J Impot Res. 2003;15:26–37.

Salonia A, Rigatti P, Montorsi F. Sildenafil in erectile dysfunction: a critical review. Curr Med Res Opin. 2003;19:241–62.

Shabsigh R, Kaufman JM, Steidle C, Padma-Nathan H. Randomized study of testosterone gel as adjunctive therapy to sildenafil in hypogonadal men with erectile dysfunction who do not respond to sildenafil alone. J Urol. 2004;172:658–63.
Traish AM, Toselli P, Jeong SJ, Kim NN. Adipocyte accumulation in penile corpus cavernosum of the orchiectomized rabbit: a potential mechanism for veno-occlusive dysfunction in androgen deficiency. J Androl. 2005;26:242–8.
Vignozzi L, Morelli A, Filippi S, et al. Testosterone regulates RhoA/Rho-kinase signaling in two distinct animal models of chemical diabetes. J Sex Med. 2007;4:620–32.
Zhang XH, Morelli A, Luconi M, et al. Testosterone regulates PDE5 expression and in vivo responsiveness to tadalafil in rat corpus cavernosum. Eur Urol. 2005;47:409–16.
Zitzmann M, Brune M, Nieschlag E. Vascular reactivity in hypogonadal men is reduced by androgen substitution. J Clin Endocrinol Metab. 2002;87:5030–7.

Chapter 11
Traditional Asian Herbs: Potential Use for Late-Onset Hypogonadism?

Peter Huat Chye Lim

Introduction

Sexual herbs throughout the ages have been eagerly consumed no matter how unappetizing or bizarre. In our never-ending search for better sex, humans have ingested such diverse items as elephant tusks, lion blood, bull testicles, rhino horn, ram penis, pig genitals, and the dried remains of the Mediterranean Cantharis beetle, otherwise known as "Spanish fly." The motivation to use these herbs has been largely to improve sexual function. Can they be used to treat hypogonadism? The Bomos (village doctors) in Malaysia and Indonesia and Chinese Traditional Medical Practitioners (in China and elsewhere) have been using these herbs for centuries. Some of these work purportedly by apparently restoring testosterone levels directly, by releasing it from testosterone-binding globulin, or by enhancing their action at the receptor sites. If these claims can be proven then surely the aging male suffering from andropause may derive benefit from their consumption. Generations of Asians taking them have either really improved physically or at least psychologically from a placebo effect. These herbals can be found throughout Asia and range from Tongkat Ali, Ginseng, to Tribulus, etc. I will discuss only

P.H.C. Lim, MBBS, MMed(Surg), M.Inst.Urol(Lon)
FAMS, D.Urol(Lon), FICS
Department of Andrology, Urology Continence Center,
Gleneagles Hospital, Singapore, Singapore

H.T. Naval Medical School, Surabaya, Indonesia

Edith Cowan University, Joondalup, WA, Australia

Society for Men's Health Singapore, Midview City, Singapore

Gleneagles Medical Centre, Singapore, Singapore

Department of Urology, Changi General Hospital, Singapore, Singapore
e-mail: tphphcl@pacific.net.sg

P.H.C. Lim (ed.), *Men's Health*,
DOI 10.1007/978-1-4471-4766-4_11,

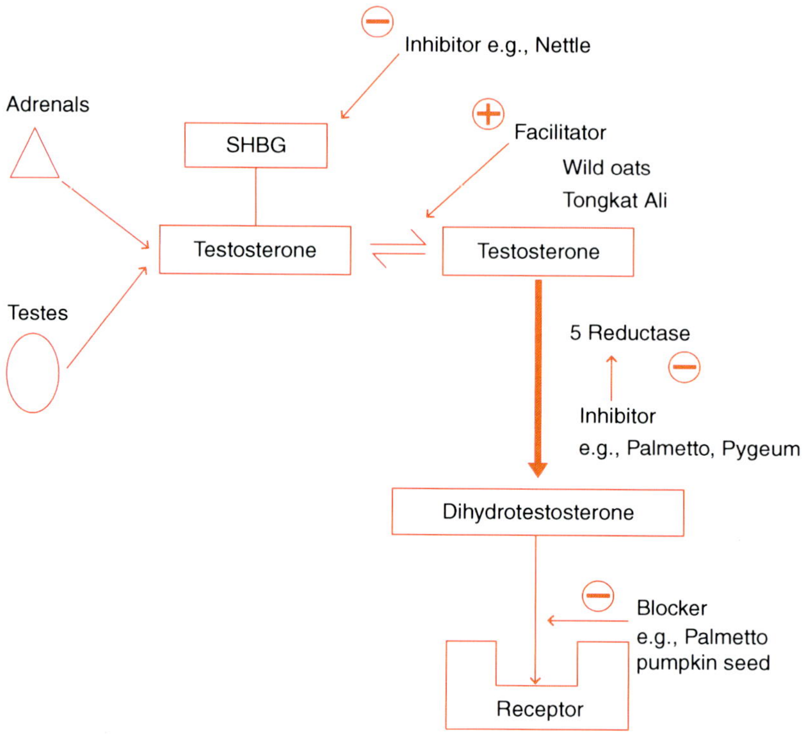

Fig. 11.1 Action sites of phytotherapies-examples

those herbs that claim to increase testosterone levels by increasing its actual level or its free fraction or cause existing testosterone to be more effective by blocking its aromatization (see Fig. 11.1).

Only the common varieties easily found ubiquitously in Asia will be covered by this author to give readers an idea of the homeopathic medical remedies used in the region.

Tribulus terrestris

This plant has long been used as a folk medicine in several parts of Asia and most widely in Eastern Europe and Bulgaria for sexual deficiency. The properties of this herb have been associated with increased sperm production, sexual endurance, and testosterone levels. Since testosterone plays a huge role for men, systemically, the use of this herb could be useful. However, it is not a hormone as some believe. In Bulgaria, the "hormone-balancing effects" of *Tribulus terrestris* are being used for premenstrual syndrome and menopausal syndrome.

There are three groups of active phytochemicals in *Tribulus terrestris*, i.e.: (1) dioscin, which may help sexual energy by increasing the free testosterone level for men and modulating pregnenolone, progesterone, estrogen, etc.; (2) sterols, this group could protect the prostate from swelling and in combination with the X steroidal saponins; and (3) steroidal saponins, which can influence the immune system and also possess antimicrobial properties (against herpes).

Tongkat Ali (Eurycoma longifolia)

This native plant found throughout Southeast Asia is used as an aphrodisiac since 1996. It has to be used regularly and apparently works by enhancing testosterone and cGMP production. Benefits are felt gradually over a period of time, mainly because it enhances the natural biological synthesis of testosterone. When this hormone level is increased, health and vitality are restored. In studies on mice, Tongkat Ali increased the frequency and duration of sexual performance by enhancing testosterone levels increasing up to 440 %. In a recent study on humans, 62 % of the subjects showed an increase of the free testosterone index indicating its possible role in the biosynthesis of steroids. Thus, its mode of action is increasing free testosterone from SHBG. It has also been shown to increase sperm concentration and motility.

Epimedium Extract (Horny Goat Weed)

The Chinese refer to this herb as "Yin Yang Huo," a "licentious goat plant"; hence, its common name is well known as "horny goat weed" in many Western cultures. Scientifically, studies have shown that Epimedium may restore low levels of both testosterone and thyroid hormone, which may account for some of its claimed benefits in improving sexual libido. It also apparently blocks conversion of testosterone into estradiol and blocks estrogen receptors in the body.

Aswaganda – 2 mode action: possibly blocks conversion of testosterone into Estradiol. The bioactive plant component also purportedly fills up and blocks estrogen receptors in the body

Pimpinella alpina (*Purwoceng*) from Java and *Lunasia amara Blanco* (*Sanrego*) from South Sulawesi in Indonesia are androgenic herbs with androgenic properties used as aphrodisiacs.

Muira Puama

The herb Ptychopetalum olacoides extracted from this is otherwise called "potency wood," and it is the best-known Amazonian folk medicine to increase libido and penile hardness. It purportedly acts as a nerve stimulant to heighten receptiveness to sexual stimuli and physical sensation of sex. Rich in sterols, e.g., sitosterol, campesterol, and lupol, it is postulated to activate the body's receptors for testosterone to heighten libido and enhance performance. Another purported action is an increase of free testosterone from its bound state to SHBG. The other ingredients present are volatile oils like camphor which are used by homeopathics to restore sex drive, inner depth of libido, and mental ability to be aroused.

Pumpkin Seed

Besides having a pleasant flavor, pumpkin seeds are known to possess antidepressant properties in Chinese history. More importantly, pumpkin seed ingestion can influence positively prostate health, which is very important for male sexual health. It is commonly used to strengthen the prostate gland and promote healthy hormone function in men. Myosin, an amino acid found in pumpkin seeds, is known to be essential for muscular contractions and increasing free testosterone from SHBG plus blocking DHT linking to DHT receptors.

Nettle Leaf

Among its many properties, nettle leaf has lately been shown to influence prostate health and prevention of prostate conditions, especially prostatitis, which is an inflammation of the prostate gland. Besides, there is also speculation that nettle leaf may help with male pattern baldness. Irrespective of the age, prostate health is essential for men. Prostate problems can interfere with a healthy sex life. Nettle is also considered to be an overall energizer of the body, as well as a natural diuretic and anti-inflammatory remedy. It is rich in iron, zinc, and chlorophyll. The claims are that it increases free testosterone from SHBG.

Ginseng (Panax Ginseng)

This is an adaptogenic herb touted to have boosted the potency of Ottoman sultans. Used to increase the body's ability to handle environmental stresses and combat biochemical imbalances, it energizes when one is fatigued and controls anxiety. It may also increase sex-related hormones like testosterone and enhances sexual responses in both sexes. It thus acts as a tonic, stimulant, and aphrodisiac. The most commonly used type is Chinese Ginseng renowned for increasing sexual vitality.

Wild Oats

Avena sativa is a biologically standardized green oats extract. A study in 1986 by the Institute for Advanced Study of Sexuality in San Francisco reported effects like heightened sexual awareness, increased sexual thoughts, more orgasms (36 % in men and 29 % in women), and some male subjects showed increased levels of testosterone attributed to unbinding of testosterone from SHBG. Oats supply steroidal saponins which modulate hormonal balance. A Singapore study done in the 1990s showed that EXSAIVA – a Swiss version of wild oats – released up to 28 % of testosterone from SHBG in a cohort of 90 volunteers tested.

Others

Saw palmetto, rye grass, Pygeum are claimed to be effective in increasing free testosterone from SHBG and inhibiting 5-alpha reductase thus preventing testosterone in becoming active DHT. Saw palmetto apparently can additionally block DHT linking to DHT receptors.

Conclusion

This chapter is intended to demonstrate the other side of medicine in Asia where use of traditional phytotherapies abounds. It serves to introduce the reader to what is essentially Asian homeopathic practices focusing on the therapies that have been claimed to increase available testosterone in the subjects using them or enhancing its utilization in the tissues by stimulatory or inhibitory bioactions. Whether these claims can be substantiated remains to be proven as few if any placebo-controlled trials have been done on them. Also the mechanism of action needs to be convincingly elucidated before the theories behind each of these herbs can be accepted as fact and not fiction. Notwithstanding the lack of complete scientific documentation, we will continue to see these herbs being used for the management of sexual hypofunction and currently for late-onset hypogonadism generated by a burgeoning interest in using testosterone replacement therapy in the aging male in Asia.

Bibliography

Ang HH, Cheang HS, Yusof AP. Effects of Eurycoma longifolia J (Tongkat Ali) on the initiation of sexual performance of inexperienced castrated male rats. Exp Anim. 2000;49:35–8.

Benny Tan KH, Victor Ong YC, Peter Lim HC. Chapter 10: Singapore experience. In: Park NC, et al, editors. Modern oriental phytotherapy in sexual medicine EDS. Publ Koon Ja Publishing Inc; 2010. p. 111–132. ISBN 978-89-6278-304-9.

Bucci LR. Selected herbals and human exercise performance. Am J Clin Nutr. 2000;72: 624S–36S.
Carey MP, Johnson BT. Effectiveness of yohimbine in the treatment of erectile disorder: Four meta-analytic integrations. Arch Sex Behav. 1996;25:341–60.
CHEMEXCIL. Tribulus terrestris L. (N.O. Zygophyllaceae). Selected medicinal plants of India. A monograph of identity, safety and clinical usage. Bombay: Tata Press; 1992. p. 323–6.
Ernst E. The desktop guide to complementary and alternative medicine – an evidence-based approach. St Louis: Mosby; 2001.
Garg SK. Evaluation of safety & efficacy of "Tentax Royal" in management of ED. Med Update. 2004;12(8):51–5.
Hryb DJ, Kahn MS, Romas NA, Rosner W. The effect of extracts of the roots of the stinging nettle (Urtica dioica) on the interaction of SHBG with its receptor on human prostatic membranes. Planta Med. 1995;61:31–2.
Komesaroff PA, Black CV, Cable V, Sudhir K. Effects of wild yam extract on menopausal symptoms, lipids and sex hormones in healthy menopausal women. Climacteric. 2001;4:144–50.
Kuang AK, Chen JL, Chen MD. Effects of yang-restoring herb medicines on the levels of plasma corticosterone, testosterone and triiodothyronine. Zhong Xi Yi Jie He Za Zhi. 1989;9:737–8. 710.
Liang P, Li H, Peng X, Jiao J, Liu J, Ye Z. Effects of Astragalus membranaceus injection on sperm abnormality in Cd-induced rats. Zhonghua Nan Ke Xue. 2004;10:42–5,48.21.
Lim PHC. Traditional Asian folklore medicines in sexual health. Indian J Urol 2006;22:241–5; 5th World Congress on the Aging male 9–12 Feb 2006, Salzburg, Austra.
Malo AF, Roldan EF, Garde J, Soler AJ, Gomendio M. Antlers honestly advertise sperm production and quality. Proc Biol Sci. 2005;272:149–57.
Meletis CD. Better sex naturally. Dean of Medical Affairs, Chief Medical Officer, National College of Naturopathic Medicine.
Natural Medicines Comprehensive Database. Compiled by the Editors of Prescriber's Letter and Pharmacist's Letter.
Natural Medicines Comprehensive Database. http://www.naturaldatabase.com/pda.
PDR Herbal and Nutritional Supplement editions. 2002, 2003.
Rowland DL, Tai W. A review of plant-derived and herbal approaches to the treatment of sexual dysfunctions. J Sex Marital Ther. 2003;29:185–205.
Wang KY, Dahlen M. Chinese herbal medicine. Hong Kong: Workman Press; 1994.
Wong KY, Daylen M. Chinese Herbal Medicines-60 Common Herbs: Principles and Practice. Hong Kong: Wokman Press 1994/1999. ISBN 962-7316-02-4.
Wong K-Y, Martha D. Chinese herbal medicine. Hong Kong: Publ Wokman Press; 1999. ISBN 962-7316-02-4.
Zhu J, Halpern G, Jones K. The scientific rediscovery of a precious ancient Chinese herbal regimen: Cordyceps sinensis: part II. J Alternat Complement Med. 1998;4:429–57.

Chapter 12
Effects of Excessive Androgen Use and Abuse

Peter Huat Chye Lim

Introduction

The main area of abuse is in bodybuilding and sports. Because androgens have other actions on the body, one particular systemic action has been exploited to good and bad use, i.e., its maintenance of muscle strength and mass. This benefit to health and QOL is useful to prevent frailty of aging but is often abused in competitive sports.

Androgenic Derivatives

The natural androgens found in the body are:

- DHEA, DHEA(S)
- Testosterone
- Dihydrotestosterone (DHT)
- Androstenedione
- Androstenediol

P.H.C. Lim, MBBS, MMed(Surg), M.Inst.Urol(Lon)
FAMS, D.Urol(Lon), FICS
Department of Andrology, Urology Continence Center,
Gleneagles Hospital, Singapore, Singapore

H.T. Naval Medical School, Surabaya, Indonesia

Edith Cowan University, Joondalup, WA, Australia

Society for Men's Health Singapore, Midview City, Singapore

Gleneagles Medical Centre, Singapore, Singapore

Department of Urology, Changi General Hospital, Singapore, Singapore
e-mail: tphphcl@pacific.net.sg

P.H.C. Lim (ed.), *Men's Health*,
DOI 10.1007/978-1-4471-4766-4_12,

Modifications to the androgen molecule which are useful to increase muscle mass are:

1. Stanozolol
    - This is a derivative of DHT which is not capable of converting into estrogen.
    - Together with a rich protein diet, muscles become leaner and harder – hence, it is popular for speed-/strength-related sports enhancing.
2. Nandrolone Decanoate
    - This is a long-acting (three weekly) version which increases muscle and lean body weight.
    - It has minimal androgenic/estrogenic properties – hence, concomitant use of a an antiandrogenic is rarely needed.
3. Oxandrolone
    - Mild androgen promotes strength and muscle hardness and reduces visceral/abdominal fat.
    - It will not aromatize; women tolerate it at low doses; it is suitable for over 40s.
    - No need for tamoxifen/clomiphene/HCG.

Undesirable Effects

Several undesirable effects may occur and these pertain to unwanted cosmetic changes, proneness to musculoskeletal injuries, male infertility due to testicular suppression, liver toxicity in those with fatty change in the liver or preexisting hepatitis, slight potential for prostate hypertrophy in a minority of men with family history of BPH, and a remote possibility of cardiac and CNS ischemic sequelae in those with preexisting heart or cerebrovascular disease. The greatest abuse seen in practice is the ubiquitous use in young men of childbearing age without forethought concerning their fertility. Testicular atrophy and azoospermia leading to subfertility and infertility rapidly ensues often by the end of 1 year.

Physical Appearance

The physical changes of the patient abusing androgens have the characteristic oily skin and acne ± scarring due to acne. Increased body hair/male pattern baldness may be demonstrable and breast enlargement (men); shrinkage (women) may be observable. In younger men premature closure of growth plates of long bones makes them shorter in stature.

Muscle and Bone Injuries

Because of the increased power in their muscles, there may be overconfidence in the amount of force used resulting in tendon rupture risks and damage to ligaments during sports. The cause is clearly the muscle force exerted exceeded the strength of the attachment to the bone.

Infertility

Special mention is required in this aspect. The risk increases with prolonged use at higher dosages. Testicular atrophy results and there may be diminished sex drive with prolonged use. It starts happening usually after 6 months of use and becomes established by 1 year.

Heart Disease

Among problems reported are falls in HDL-C lipoproteins (recovers after 1-month cessation), glucose intolerance, increased insulin resistance with some anabolic steroids, and cardiomegaly with ejection fraction <40 %.

Stroke (CVA)

Reports have been received of CVA's with use of abnormally high doses with thrombotic strokes developing.

Prostate Disease

There is a slight potential for prostate hypertrophy (BPH) in a minority of men with family history of BPH. Slight increases of prostate volume and slight decreases of uroflow rates are not uncommon, but these are small changes which plateau off in the vast majority of men treated. Slight increases of PSA have been noted but again they tend to plateau off. The chance of getting cancer of the prostate is today considered remote as men with low levels of testosterone are currently deemed at greater risk of cancer (Morgentaler, 2003–2008).

Liver Disease and Cancer

There is a very strong negative effect on the liver especially with the older generation of androgens, especially the 17 alpha-alkylated steroids. Notorious is the methylated version, and it is well documented that methyltestosterone causes obstructive type jaundice. Peliosis hepatis can occur but a rarer complication is the development of liver tumors; risk is higher with very long-term use. In woman-to-man sex change patients with years and years of the older types of testosterone being injected, we have seen liver tumors occurring not infrequently.

Psychological Effects

Often referred to as the "testosterone rage." There may be increased aggression – criminal acts of violence vs. people and property and fits of recklessness. This "roid rage" – highly aggressive out-of-control behavior – occurs in <1 % of men abusing themselves with testosterone for enhancement. The role of previous mental illness or abuse of other drugs may be highly contributory. Some men continue to request for treatment not because they actually need it but because of a possible placebo effect. Other modes of presentation are psychosis and depression.

User Dependence

The development of physical dependence is a real potential problem and psychological dependence develops in 25–50 %.

Women and Steroids

In women, there is the problem of masculinization – loss of scalp hair, growth of facial hair, spread of pubic hair, deepening of voice, and enlargement of clitoris (mostly permanent). Other problems include acne, increased aggression, liver and cholesterol changes (reversible), decrease in breast size, menstrual changes – leading to cessation or lighter flow and difficulty to conceive as the main complaints. There is also the possibility of birth defects of babies born and polycystic ovaries developing.

Bibliography

Achar S, Rostamian A, Narayan SM. Cardiac and metabolic effects of anabolic-androgenic steroid abuse on lipids, blood pressure, left ventricular dimensions, and rhythm. Am J Cardiol. 2010;106(6):893–901.

Arnold AM, Peralta JM, Thonney ML. Ontogeny of growth hormone, insulin-like growth factor-I, estradiol and cortisol in the growing lamb: effect of testosterone. J Endocrinol. 1996;150(3):391–9.

Baggish AL, Weiner RB, Kanayama G, Hudson JI, Picard MH, Hutter Jr AM, et al. Long-term anabolic-androgenic steroid use is associated with left ventricular dysfunction. Circ Heart Fail. 2010;3(4):472–6.

Bahrke MS, Yesalis 3rd CE, Wright JE. Psychological and behavioural effects of endogenous testosterone levels and anabolic-androgenic steroids among males. A review. Sports Med. 1990;10(5):303–37.

Basaria S. Androgen abuse in athletes: detection and consequences. J Clin Endocrinol Metab. 2010;95(4):1533–43.

Basaria S, Wahlstrom JT, Dobs AS. Clinical review 138: anabolic-androgenic steroid therapy in the treatment of chronic diseases. J Clin Endocrinol Metab. 2001;86(11):5108–17.

Berger JR, Pall L, Hall CD, et al. Oxandrolone in AIDS-wasting myopathy. AIDS. 1996;10(14): 1657–62.

Berkow R, editor. The Merck manual of diagnosis and therapy. 15th ed. Rahway: Merck Sharp and Dohme Research Laboratories; 1987. p. 1208.

Birgner C, Kindlundh-Högberg AM, Alsiö J, et al. The anabolic androgenic steroid nandrolone decanoate affects mRNA expression of dopaminergic but not serotonergic receptors. Brain Res. 2008;1240:221–8.

Bucher G, Berger DS, Fields-Gardner C, et al. A prospective study on the safety and effect of nandrolone decanoate in HIV positive patients. In: Abstract of the 11th Conference on AIDS, Vancouver, 1996.

Danhaive PA, Rousseau GG. Binding of glucocorticoid antagonists to androgen and glucocorticoid hormone receptors in rat skeletal muscle. J Steroid Biochem. 1986;24(2):481–7.

Demling R, De Santi L. Closure of the "non-healing wound" corresponds with correction of weight loss using the anabolic agent oxandrolone. Ostomy Wound Manage. 1998;44(10):58–62, 64, 66 passim.

Di Paolo M, Agozzino M, Toni C, et al. Sudden anabolic steroid abuse-related death in athletes. Int J Cardiol. 2007;114(1):114–7. Epub 2005 Dec 20.

Di Pasquale MG. Drug Use and detection in amateur sports. Warkworth: MGD Press; 1984.

Dimick DF, Heron M, Baulieu EE, et al. A comparative study of the metabolic fate of testosterone, 17 alpha-methyl-testosterone. 19-nor-testosterone. 17 alpha-methyl-19-nor-testosterone and 17 alpha-methylestr-5(10)-ene-17 beta-ol-3-one in normal males. Clin Chim Acta. 1961;6: 63–71.

Falanga V, Greenberg AS, Zhou L, et al. Stimulation of collagen synthesis by the anabolic steroid stanozolol. J Invest Dermatol. 1998;111(6):1193–7.

Ferreira IM, Verreschi IT, Nery LE, et al. The influence of 6 months of oral anabolic steroids on body mass and respiratory muscles in undernourished COPD patients. Chest. 1998;114(1):19–28.

Fineschi V, Riezzo I, Centini F, et al. Sudden cardiac death during anabolic steroid abuse: morphologic and toxicologic findings in two fatal cases of bodybuilders. Int J Legal Med. 2007;121(1):48–53. Epub 2005 Nov 15.

Gaughan WJ, Liss KA, Dunn SR, et al. A 6-month study of low-dose recombinant human erythropoietin alone and in combination with androgens for the treatment of anemia in chronic hemodialysis patients. Am J Kidney Dis. 1997;30(4):495–500.

Gaul, Morato, Hayano, et al. Biosynthesis of estrogens. Endocrinol. 1962;71.

Gold J, High HA, Li Y, et al. Safety and efficacy of nandrolone decanoate for treatment of wasting in patients with HIV infection. AIDS. 1996;10(7):745–52.

Graham MR, Evans P, Davies B, Baker JS. AAS, growth hormone, and insulin abuse: psychological and neuroendocrine effects. Ther Clin Risk Manag. 2008;4(3):587–97.

Johansen KL, Mulligan K, Schambelan M. Anabolic effects of nandrolone decanoate in patients receiving dialysis: a randomized controlled trial. JAMA. 1999;281(14):1275–81.

Kokkevi A, Fotiou A, Chileva A, et al. Daily exercise and anabolic steroids use in adolescents: a cross-national European study. Subst Use Misuse. 2008;43(14):2053–65.

Lau DH, Stiles MK, John B, et al. Atrial fibrillation and anabolic steroid abuse. Int J Cardiol. 2007;117(2):e86–7.

Mendenhall CL, Moritz TE, Roselle GA, et al. A study of oral nutritional support with oxandrolone in malnourished patients with alcoholic hepatitis: results of a Department of Veterans Affairs cooperative study. Hepatology. 1993;17(4):564–76.

Phillis BD, Abeywardena MY, Adams MJ, et al. Nandrolone potentiates arrhythmogenic effects of cardiac ischemia in the rat. Toxicol Sci. 2007;99(2):605–11. Epub 2007 Jul 25.

Rada RT, Kellner R, Winslow WW. Plasma testosterone and aggressive behavior. Psychosomatics. 1976;17(3):138–42.

Rosenfeld RL. Role of androgens in growth and development of the fetus, child, and adolescent. Adv Pediatr. 1972;19:171–213.

Samuels LT, Sellers DM, McCaulay CJ. The source of excess creatine following methyl testosterone. J Clin Endocrinol Metab. 1946;6(10):655–63.

Schols AM, Soeters PB, Mostert R, et al. Physiologic effects of nutritional support and anabolic steroids in patients with chronic obstructive pulmonary disease. A placebo-controlled randomized trial. Am J Respir Crit Care Med. 1995;152(4 Pt 1):1268–74.

Schwingel PA, Cotrim HP, Salles BR, Almeida CE, dos Santos Jr CR, Nachef B, et al. Anabolic-androgenic steroids: a possible new risk factor of toxicant-associated fatty liver disease. Liver Int. 2011;31(3):348–53.

Snyder PJ, Peachey H, Hannoush P, et al. Effect of testosterone treatment on bone mineral density in men over 65 years of age. J Clin Endocrinol Metab. 1999;84(6):1966–72.

Spungen AM, Grimm DR, Strakhan M, et al. Treatment with an anabolic agent is associated with improvement in respiratory function in persons with tetraplegia: a pilot study. Mt Sinai J Med. 1999;66(3):201–5.

Steele RE, Didato F, Steinetz BG. Relative importance of 5alpha reduction for the androgenic and LH-inhibiting activities of delta-4-3-ketosteroids. Steroids. 1977;29(3):331–48.

Strawford A, Barbieri T, Van Loan M, et al. Resistance exercise and supraphysiologic androgen therapy in eugonadal men with HIV-related weight loss: a randomized controlled trial. JAMA. 1999;281(14):1282–90.

Talih F, Fattal O, Malone Jr D. Anabolic steroid abuse: psychiatric and physical costs. Cleve Clin J Med. 2007;74(5):341–4, 346, 349–52.

Urban RJ, Bodenburg YH, Gilkison C, et al. Testosterone administration to elderly men increases skeletal muscle strength and protein synthesis. Am J Physiol. 1995;269(5 Pt 1):E820–6.

Vogel W, Klaiber EL, Broverman DM. A comparison of the antidepressant effects of a synthetic androgen (mesterolone) and amitriptyline in depressed men. J Clin Psychiatry. 1985;46(1):6–8.

Wilson IC, Prange Jr AJ, Lara PP. Methyltestosterone with imipramine in men: conversion of depression to paranoid reaction. Am J Psychiatry. 1974;131(1):21–4.

Chapter 13
Practice Pointers for the Practitioner

Peter Huat Chye Lim

Testosterone Lozenges/Troches

Each Striant™ lozenge (buccal system) comes in a blister pack. The lozenge must be kept in the blister pack until ready for use.

- Use: The lozenge has one flat side and one round side. The round side goes against the gums. The flat side goes against the cheek.
- When ready, put a lozenge in the mouth, start by putting the flat side of the lozenge on the fingertip. Place the lozenge up against the gums and to the left or right of the two front teeth. Gently push the lozenge up as high as it will go onto the gum. Take the finger out of the mouth and push on the lozenge from the outside of your upper lip for at least 30 s. The lozenge should stick to the gum. It is okay if it sticks to the cheek instead of the gum.
- Do not chew or swallow the lozenge.
- Each time a new lozenge is used, put it on the side opposite from where the last lozenge was placed. If the morning lozenge was on the right side, put the evening lozenge on the left side.
- The lozenge will stay in the mouth all the time. It will get softer and slowly melt, but will not melt completely. It has to be removed after 12 h. Use the finger to gently loosen the lozenge. Then carefully slide it down along the tooth and take it out of the mouth.

P.H.C. Lim, MBBS, MMed(Surg), M.Inst.Urol(Lon)
FAMS, D.Urol(Lon), FICS
Department of Andrology, Urology Continence Center,
Gleneagles Hospital, Singapore, Singapore

H.T. Naval Medical School, Surabaya, Indonesia

Edith Cowan University, Joondalup, WA, Australia

Society for Men's Health Singapore, Midview City, Singapore

Gleneagles Medical Centre, Singapore, Singapore

Department of Urology, Changi General Hospital, Singapore, Singapore
e-mail: tphphcl@pacific.net.sg

P.H.C. Lim (ed.), *Men's Health*,
DOI 10.1007/978-1-4471-4766-4_13,

- Unless changing lozenges, keep the lozenge in the mouth when eating or brushing the teeth. After eating or brushing the teeth, check to make sure the lozenge is still in place.
- Usual dose is two times a day, once in the morning and once in the evening (about 12 h apart). It may be easiest to put the lozenge on the gums after having eaten breakfast and brushing the teeth and after you have eaten the evening meal.

Testosterone Cream and Gel

- Topical testosterone avoids the need for injections or patches and may reduce the large variation in blood level of standard injectable testosterone, which is commonly given once every 2 weeks. However, the drug supplied by the cream or gel has a much shorter half-life in the body, so it is usually applied twice a day.
- Available as cream or gel form, in any concentration from 1 to 100 mg/g (some pharmacies indicate concentration in percent; 100 mg/g is 10 % testosterone). A 1-month supply usually contains 60 g of cream or gel. It comes with a measuring device and instructions on applying 1 g twice per day.
- Older men who are being treated for hypogonadism usually use the 25 mg/g strength twice daily (cf women use much lower doses, usually the 2–5 mg/g concentrations twice daily).
- The gel is alcohol based.
- The usual amount of the cream or gel applied is 1 g twice per day. Men can also apply it to the scrotum, because absorption may be better there since the skin is thin.

Testosterone Pellet Therapy

- Advantage is infrequent dosing and typically pellets are implanted every 3–4 months. The dosing is smooth and steady and there are fewer side effects. Unlike other methods, they release small amounts of T into the blood stream, which mimic the body's own T production. This eliminates the erratic swings in T levels that come along with other forms of testosterone therapy traditional delivery methods. This greatly reduces the occurrence of side effects.
- The disadvantages are as follows: (1) minor surgery is required to implant the pellets; (2) there may be some minor pain, especially the day after implantation; and (3) on rare occasions, the implants can resurface and come out of the skin.

Methods of Implantation of Testosterone Pellets

- The implant procedure consists of a small incision through which a narrow cannula is inserted.
- The pellets are inserted through the cannula, then the cannula is withdrawn.

- The incision is then closed with a Steri-Strip or stitch, and pressure is applied until bleeding stops. The area is then covered with a dressing.

Oral Testosterone Capsules (Andriol)

Andriol Testocaps must be taken with a meal which should contain some fat. Swallow the capsules whole without chewing, using some water or other fluid. Take half of the daily dose in the morning and the other half in the evening. If the daily dose is an uneven number of capsules, take the larger number in the morning. The usual dosage is 3–4 capsules daily during the first 2–3 weeks, followed by a gradual decrease to 1–3 capsules daily if needed.

Three Monthly Depot Testosterone Injections (Nebido)

Nebido Injection Technique

- Inform patient: expect some pain/discomfort at injection site – few hours.
- Warm up ampoule in your hands.
- Draw out using 19-G needle, inject using 21-G needle (green).
- Deep IM injection over *upper outer quadrant of buttock.*
- Administer over *2–3 min.*
- Encourage ambulation thereafter.

Immediate Adverse Effects

- Pain at injection site
- Sensation of warmth, flushing
  - Brief
  - Can be minimized by giving over 3–4 min (i.e., very slowly)
- Cough, "choking" sensation (vasovagal)
  - Brief
  - Can be minimized by giving over 3–4 min (i.e., very slowly)

Chapter 14
Collection Charts/Questionnaires/Testosterone Calculators/Other Aide-Memoires, etc. for the GP

Peter Huat Chye Lim

- Erectile function (six questions, score range 1–30)
- Orgasmic function (two questions, score range 0–10)
- Sexual desire (two questions, score range 2–10)
- Intercourse satisfaction (three questions, score range 0–15)
- Overall satisfaction (two questions, score range 2–10)

Total Testosterone

Total Testosterone = free Testosterone + Alb-bound Testosterone + SHBG-bound Testosterone

Bioavailable Testosterone

Bio Testosterone = Albumin-bound Testosterone + SHBG-bound Testosterone

P.H.C. Lim, MBBS, MMed(Surg), M.Inst.Urol(Lon)
FAMS, D.Urol(Lon), FICS
Department of Andrology, Urology Continence Cenmter,
Gleneagles Hospital, Singapore, Singapore

H.T. Naval Medical School, Surabaya, Indonesia

Edith Cowan University, Joondalup, WA, Australia

Society for Men's Health Singapore, Midview City, Singapore

Gleneagles Medical Centre, Singapore, Singapore

Department of Urology, Changi General Hospital, Singapore, Singapore
e-mail: tphphcl@pacific.net.sg

P.H.C. Lim (ed.), *Men's Health*,
DOI 10.1007/978-1-4471-4766-4_14,

SHBG

Total SHBG = free SHBG + steroid-bound SHBG or free SHBG = total SHBG− steroid-bound SHBG (Vermeulen etal. 1999).

WHO Definition of the Metabolic Syndrome in Men

- Hyperinsulinemia (upper quartile of the nondiabetic population) or fasting plasma glucose ≥110 mg/dL
  - AND at least two of the following:
- Abdominal obesity
  - Definition 1: waist-hip ratio > 0.90 or BMI ≥30
  - Definition 2: waist girth ≥94 cm
- Dyslipidemia (serum triglycerides ≥150 mg/dL or HDL cholesterol < 35 mg /dL)
- Hypertension (blood pressure ≥140/90 mmHg or medication) (Balkau et al. 1999)

Recent Guidelines

Recent publication of two major sets of guidelines have provided some clarity when making a diagnosis.

There are no generally accepted lower limits of normal and it is unclear whether geographically different thresholds depend on ethnic differences or on the physician's perception.

However, there is general agreement that total testosterone (TT) above 12 nmol/L (346 ng/dL) or free Testosterone above 250 pmol/L (72 pg/mL) does not require substitution.

Total testosterone below 8 nmol/L (231 ng/dL) or free Testosterone below 180 pmol/L (52 pg/mL) requires substitution.

In symptomatic men with total testosterone levels between 8 and 12 nmol/L, a trial of testosterone therapy can be considered.

Which of the following symptoms apply to you at this time? Please, mark the approprite box each symptom. For symptoms that do not apply, please mark "none".

Symptoms:	None	Mild	Moderate	Severe	Extremely severe	
Score =	1	2	3	4	5	**Ageing Male Symptom(AMS) score**
1. **Decline in your feeing of general well-being** (general state of health, subjective feeling)	☐	☐	☐	☐	☐	
2. **Joint pain and muscular ache** (lower back pain, joint pain, pain in a limb, general back ache)	☐	☐	☐	☐	☐	
3. **Excessive sweating** (unexpected/sudden episodes of sweating, hot flushes independent of strain)	☐	☐	☐	☐	☐	**Assesses sexual, psychological & somatic complaints**
4. **Sleep problems** (difficulty in falling a sleep, difficulty in sleeping through, waking up early and feeling tired, poor sleep, sleeplessness)	☐	☐	☐	☐	☐	
5. **Increased need for sleep, often feeling tired**	☐	☐	☐	☐	☐	
6. **Irritability** (feeing aggressive, easily upset about little things, moody)	☐	☐	☐	☐	☐	**Severity does not necessarity correlate with testosterone level.**
7. **Nervousness** (inner tension, restlessness, feeling fidgety)	☐	☐	☐	☐	☐	
8. **Anxiety** (feeling panicky)	☐	☐	☐	☐	☐	
9. **Physical exhaustion/lacking vitality** (general decrease in performance, reduced activity, lacking interest in leisure activities, feeling of getting less done, of achieving less, of having to force oneself to undertake activities)	☐	☐	☐	☐	☐	**No single symptom pathonomonic of hypogonadism**
10. **Decrease in muscular strength** (feeling of weakness)	☐	☐	☐	☐	☐	
11. **Depressive mood** (feeling down, sad, on the verge of tears, lack of drive, mood swings, feeing nothing is of any use)	☐	☐	☐	☐	☐	
12. **Feeling that you have passed your peak**	☐	☐	☐	☐	☐	
13. **Feeling burnt out, having hit rock-bottom**	☐	☐	☐	☐	☐	
14. **Decrease in beard growth**	☐	☐	☐	☐	☐	**www.issam.ch**
15. **Decrease in ability/frequency to perform sexually**	☐	☐	☐	☐	☐	
16. **Decrease in thenumber of morning erections**	☐	☐	☐	☐	☐	
17. **Decrease in sexual desire/libido** (lacking pleasure in sex, lacking desire for sexual intercours	☐	☐	☐	☐	☐	
Have you got any other major symptoms?	Yes	☐	No	☐		
If Yes, please describe:						

Fig. 14.1 Aging male (AMS) symptom score questionnare (Heinemann et al. 2003)

Endocrine Society Clinical Practice Guidelines 2006

Monitoring Strategies and Schedule

- We recommend evaluating the patient 3 months after treatment initiation and then annually to assess whether symptoms have responded to treatment and whether the patient is suffering any adverse effects.
- We suggest monitoring testosterone levels 3 months after initiation of testosterone therapy.
- We recommend determining hematocrit at baseline, at 3 months and then annually. If hematocrit is greater than 54 %, stop therapy until hematocrit decreases to a safe level.
- We recommend digital examination of the prostate and PSA measurement before initiating treatment, at 3 months and then in accordance with evidence-based guidelines for prostate cancer screening, depending on the age and race of the patient (Bhasin et al. 2006).

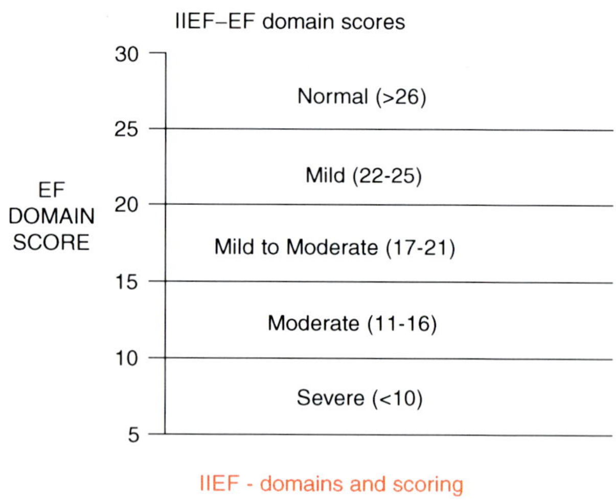

Fig. 14.2 IIEF-EF domain scores in relation to degree of ED (Cappelleri et al. 1999)

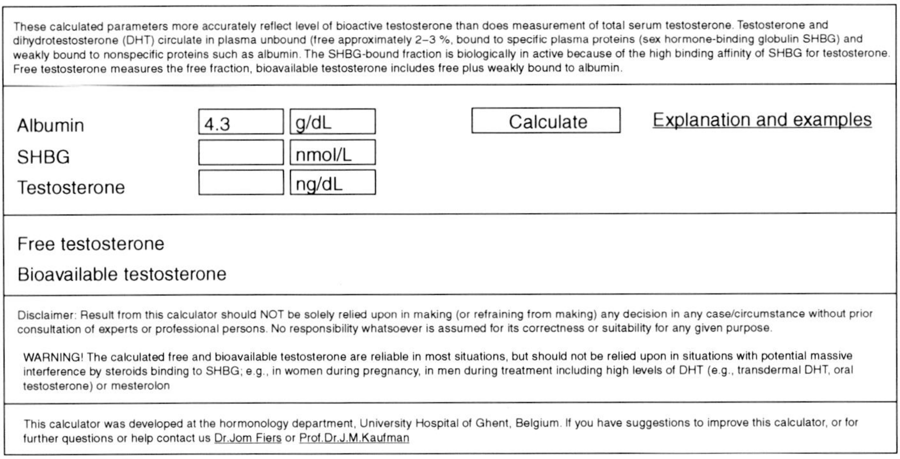

Fig. 14.3 Free testosterone calculator on interational society for study of the aging male website

References

Balkau B, Charles MA. Comment on the provisional report from the WHO consultation. European Study Group for the Study of Insulin Resistance (EGIR). Diabet Med. 1999;16:442–3.

Bhasin S, et al. Testosterone therapy in adult men with androgen deficiency syndromes: an endocrine society clinical practice guideline. J Clin Endocrinol Metab. 2006;91(6):1995–2010.

Cappelleri JC, Rosen RC, Smith MD, et al. Diagnostic evaluation of the erectile function domain of the International Index of Erectile Function. Urology. 1999;54:346–51. [PubMed].

Heinemann LAJ, Farid S et al. The Aging Males' Symptoms (AMS) scale: Update and compilation of international versions in Health Qual Life Outcomes. 2003;1:15.

Vermeulen A, Verdonck L, Kaufman JM. A critical evaluation of simple methods for the estimation of free testosterone in serum. J Clin Endocrinol Metab. 1999;84:3666–72.

Part II
Premature Ejaculation

Chapter 15
Introduction

Peter Huat Chye Lim

Definition

Premature ejaculation (*PE*) is a condition where a man ejaculates earlier than he or his partner would like him to. Premature ejaculation is also known as *rapid ejaculation*, *rapid climax*, *premature climax*, or *early ejaculation*.

Masters and Johnson define PE as occurring when a man ejaculates before his sex partner achieves orgasm, in more than 50 % of their sexual encounters. Others defined premature ejaculation as occurring if the man ejaculates within 2 min of penetration; however, Lue et al. (2004) demonstrated that three quarters of men ejaculate within 2 min of penetration in over half of their sexual encounters. Self-reported surveys report up to 75 % of men ejaculate within 10 min of penetration.

Essential criteria for making the diagnosis include:

1. Brief ejaculatory latency
2. Loss of control
3. Psychological distress in patient and/or partner

Classification: (1) primary (lifelong) and (2) secondary (acquired)

P.H.C. Lim, MBBS, MMed(Surg), M.Inst.Urol(Lon)
FAMS, D.Urol(Lon), FICS
Department of Andrology, Urology Continence Centre, Gleneagles Hospital, Singapore, Singapore

H.T. Naval Medical School, Surabaya, Indonesia

Edith Cowan University, Joondalup, WA, Australia

Society for Men's Health Singapore, Midview City, Singapore

Gleneagles Medical Centre, Singapore, Singapore

Department of Urology, Changi General Hospital, Singapore, Singapore
e-mail: tphphcl@pacific.net.sg

P.H.C. Lim (ed.), *Men's Health*,
DOI 10.1007/978-1-4471-4766-4_15,

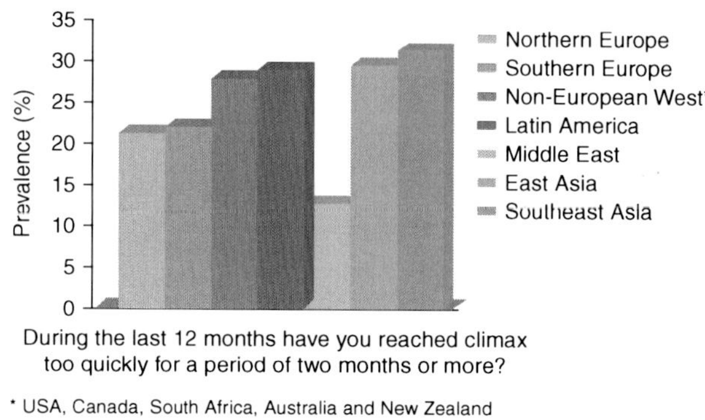

Fig. 15.1 PE is a global problem: overall PE prevalence by region (Nicolosi et al. 2004)

Epidemiology

PE is one of the most common male sexual disorders affecting 20–30 % of men. Thirty percent men with PE have concomitant ED (Janninib and Lenzi 2005; Wang et al. 2006; Lue et al. 2004) (Fig. 15.1). Most men experience premature ejaculation at least once in their lives. PE affects 25–40 % of men in the United States. Current evidence supports an average intravaginal ejaculation latency time (IELT) of 6½ min in 18–30 year olds (Ejaculation delay: what's normal? 2005; Waldinger et al. 2005a). If an IELT percentile below 2.5 is used, then premature ejaculation could be suggested by an IELT of less than about 1½ min (Waldinger et al. 2005b). However, we know that men with IELTs below 1.5 min could be "happy" and may not complain, while a man with 2-min IELT may have the perception of poor control over his ejaculation, is distressed, has interpersonal difficulties, and therefore be diagnosed with PE.

Singapore (Prevalence Study Data On File 2010)

A survey of PE in Singapore was conducted between February 6 and March 2010. The method used was via an in-person, multilocation, and online survey involving 243 patients. Breakdown by age groups is as follows:

18–35 years old: 96 (40 %)
36–45 years old: 83 (34 %)
46–55 years old: 64 (26 %)

All respondents were asked five questions about ejaculation. Each question has five possible answers, with a number (0–4) assigned to each answer.

- How difficult is it for you to delay ejaculation?
- Do you ejaculate before you want to?
- Do you ejaculate with very little stimulation?
- Do you feel frustrated because of ejaculating before you want to?

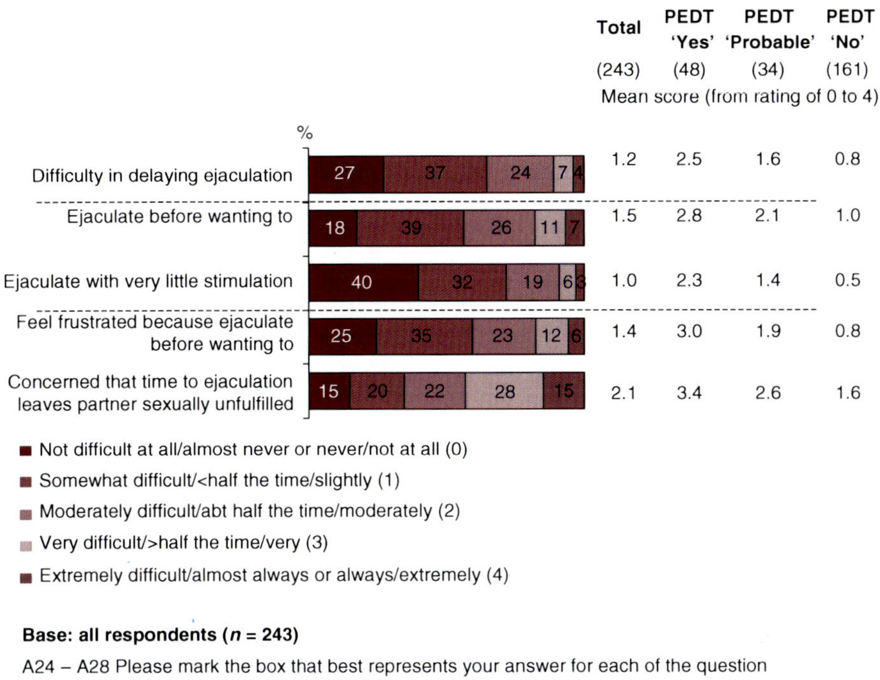

Fig. 15.2 Prevalence of PE from premature ejaculation diagnostic tool (PEDT tool)

- How concerned are you that your time of ejaculation leaves your partner sexually unfulfilled?
- A PEDT score is obtained by adding the total numbers of these five questions. A respondent is diagnosed to be with or without PE by:

  PEDT score ≥ 11: With PE
  PEDT score = 9 or 10: Probable PE
  PEDT score ≤ 8: No PE

The prevalence of PE was examined in three ways, through a validated diagnostic PE tool (PEDT), through an index, and through self-assessment (Fig. 15.2). The PEDT shows that about 20 % of the respondents have PE and about 14 % of them "probably" have PE (Fig. 15.3). The numbers coincide with the Index of Premature Ejaculation. Almost 34 % of the respondents interviewed did not have control over when they ejaculated, which led to high levels of dissatisfaction. These numbers again confirmed as almost 38 % of the respondents who had sexual intercourse over the last 1 month were extremely distressed about their control over ejaculation. When asked to self-diagnose, 16 % of the respondents felt that they definitely have PE and of the total, 31 % of them felt that they ejaculated too soon. The conclusion is that nearly 30 % of the men in Singapore have some form of PE which converts to almost half a million of potential patients with PE (Prevalence Study Data On File 2010).

- Among respondents diagnosed with PE, at least 79 % feel frustrated due to ejaculation before wanting to and 92 % feel concerned that time to ejaculation leaves partner sexually unfulfilled.

	All respondents (243)	PEDT 'Yes' (48)	PEDT 'Probable' (34)	PEDT 'No' (161)
	% of respondents who answered 'very difficult' or 'extremely difficult'			
Difficulty in delaying ejaculation	12 %	52 %	3 %	1 %
	% of respondents who answered 'more than half the time' or 'almost always or always'			
Ejaculate before wanting to	18 %	60 %	26 %	3 %
Ejaculate with very little stimulation	9 %	38 %	9 %	1 %
	% of respondents who answered 'very' or 'extremely'			
Feel frustrated because ejaculate before wanting to	18 %	79 %	6 %	2 %
Concerned that time to ejaculation leaves partner sexually unfulfilled	43 %	92 %	47 %	28 %

Base: all respondents (*n* = 243)

A24 – A28 Please mark the box that best represents your answer for each of the question

Fig. 15.3 Prevalence of PE from premature ejaculation diagnostic tool

Malaysia

As many as one in three men in Malaysia could be suffering from premature ejaculation (PE), according to a poll done by the Asia-Pacific Premature Ejaculation Prevalence And Attitude Study which surveyed nearly 5,000 men, aged 18–65, from ten Asia-Pacific countries, including China, Australia, New Zealand, Thailand, South Korea, and Malaysia.

Adverse Effects on Sexual Function and Satisfaction

Repeated PE, particularly when the man is criticized, actively or passively, by his partner, may lead to loss of self-esteem, anxiety, ED and reduced libido. It may also lead to sexual difficulties for the partner due to lack of adequate foreplay and may contribute to anorgasmia. The presence of PE in the man may be revealed when his partner presents with sexual dysfunction.

Mainly the patient suffers from:

- Diminished satisfaction with sexual relationship
- Diminished satisfaction with sexual intercourse

- Epidemiology
  - 25.35 % (men ages 18–59 and older)*
  - Most common male sexual disorder
  - Coexists frequebtly with ED
  - Primary (lifelong) vs secondary (acquired)
  - Doesn't go away with time or sexual experiences
  - Distresses patients AND partners: affects control and satisfaction

* Laumann et al. (1999). ↑ Symonds et al. (2003). McCabe. (1997).

Fig. 15.4 Premature ejaculation prevalence: the need to diagnose and treat

- Diminished sexual arousal
- Decreased discussing of sexual problem with partner
- Increased anxiety about sexual intercourse
- Diminished chance of getting an erection

PE and Erectile Dysfunction

Premature ejaculation is often followed by ED and then by lack of sexual desire. Thirty percent of men with PE have concomitant ED. PE often occurs without full erection. When ED occurs with PE the erectile dysfunction should be treated first.

In the Spore Prevalence study done by Janssen-Cilag, the prevalence of ED was in the range of 12–23 %. When asked to judge as to which one was a greater concern, 21 % felt that PE was a bigger concern, while 19 % felt that ED was a bigger concern to them. Men thus have greater concern for PE compared to ED though both are equally a challenge.

Summary (Fig. 15.4)

PE is considered to be the most common male sexual dysfunction. There are more PE patients than the 31 million ED patients reported in the USA. In fact most of the ED patients also have PE problems (Fig. 15.5). PE is mainly underreported due to reluctance of men to acknowledge, discuss or self-report PE (Rowland 2004). Lack of doctor-directed screening for sexual health concerns contribute to this underreporting.

The prevalence of PE in Singapore calculated using the Premature Ejaculation Diagnostic Tool (PEDT) was about 20 %, and those who "probably" have PE are about 14 %. Thus about 34 % of the male respondents interviewed in Singapore have some form of PE.

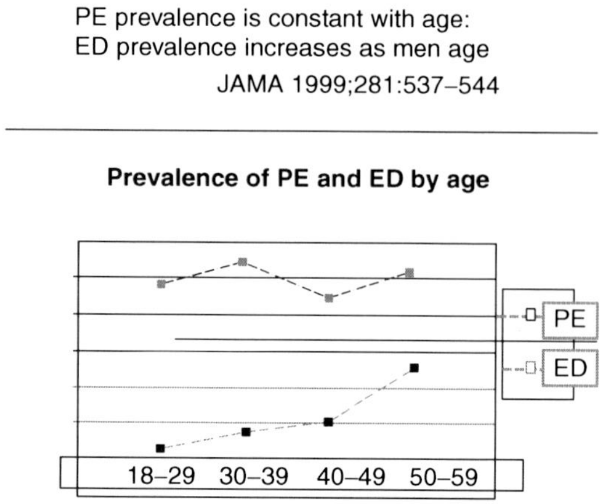

Fig. 15.5 Prevalence of ED and PE

Other than behavioral therapy and counseling, we have hitherto relied on off-label use of SSRI's and anesthetic creams as adjunctive medications for this disorder. OTC anesthetic drugs abound in the marketplace and may work but would also compromise the pleasant sexual sensation for the male partner. Hence, there is no officially licensed effective treatment available today until the launch of Dapoxetine – the only drug approved by health regulatory authorities in seven European Union countries, including Sweden, Austria, Italy, and New Zealand and South Korea. Janssen-Cilag has recently submitted Dapoxetine to the Singapore health authorities here for review and is pending approval.

References

Ejaculation delay: what's normal? [July 2005; 137–4]. http://www.medicine.ox.ac.uk/bandolier/band137/b137-4.html.

Janninib EA, Lenzi A. Epidemiology of premature ejaculation. Current Opinion in Urology. 2005;15:399–403.

Laumann EO, Paik A, Rosen RC. Sexual dysfunction in the United States: prevalence and predictors. JAMA. 1999;281:537–544.

Lue TF, Basson R, Rosen RC, et al. Sexual medicine-sexual dysfunctions in men and women. Health Publications: Paris; 2004. 9. Cited 2007;51:816–24. [PubMed]. 8.

McCabe MP. *Intimacy and quality of life among sexually dysfunctional men and women*. J Sex Marital Ther. 1997;23(4):276–90.

Nicolosi A, Laumann EO, Glasser DB, Moreira Jr ED, Paik A, Gingell C. Sexual behavior and sexual dysfunctions after age 40: the global study of sexual attitudes and behaviors. Urol. 2004;64(5):991–7.

Prevalence Study Data On File, Janssen Cilag, 2010.

Rowland DL, Perelman MA, Althof SE, Barada J, McCullough A, Bull S, et al. Self-reported premature ejaculation and aspects of sexual functioning and satisfaction. J Sex Med. 2004;1:225.

Symonds T, Roblin D, Hart K, and Althof, S. How does premature ejaculation impact a man's life? J Sex Marital Ther. 2003;29:361–70.

Waldinger MD, Quinn P, Dilleen M, Mundayat R, Schweitzer DH, Boolell M. A multinational population survey of intravaginal ejaculation latency time. The journal of sexual medicine. 2005a;2(4):492–7.

Waldinger MD, Zwinderman AH, Olivier B, Schweitzer DH. Proposal for a definition of lifelong premature ejaculation based on epidemiological stopwatch data. The journal of sexual medicine. 2005b;2(4):498–507.

Wang WF, Minhas S, Ralph DJ. Phosphodiesterase 5 inhibitors in the treatment of premature ejaculation. International J Androl. 2006;29(5):503–67.

Chapter 16
Etiology of Premature Ejaculation

Louis Gooren

The etiology of premature ejaculation is not well understood (International Society for Sexual Medicine 2008; Waldinger 2007). From an etiological and therapeutic viewpoint, it is useful to distinguish between primary (lifelong, from the onset of sexual functioning) and secondary premature ejaculation (acquired after a period of normal sexual functioning) (Sharlip 2006); the latter is not rarely associated with other sexual dysfunctions, such as erectile difficulties (Rosen 2000).

The Neurophysiological Substrate of Ejaculation

In order to understand the pathophysiology and (potential) pharmacotherapy of premature ejaculation, some insight into the neurological substrate of the process of ejaculation is desirable (Waldinger 2002; Kimura et al. 1982; Waldinger and Olivier 1998). Ejaculation involves three basic mechanisms:

- Emission
- Expulsion
- Orgasm

A schematic representation of the neurobiological substrate is presented in picture 1 (Fig. 16.1). Stimulation of the sensory receptors (Krause finger corpuscles in the mucosa of the glans penis mucosal) is relayed by the pudendal nerve afferent fibers to S4 and then to the hypogastric plexus at the T10–L2 sympathetic ganglia, whereupon this sensory information is relayed to the brain, where three ejaculatory centers are situated.

L. Gooren, M.D., Ph.D.
Department of Endocrinology, Free University of Amsterdam,
Amsterdam, the Netherlands

H.T. Naval Medical School,
Surabaya, Indonesia
e-mail: louisjgooren@gmail.com

P.H.C. Lim (ed.), *Men's Health*,
DOI 10.1007/978-1-4471-4766-4_16, © Springer-Verlag London 2013

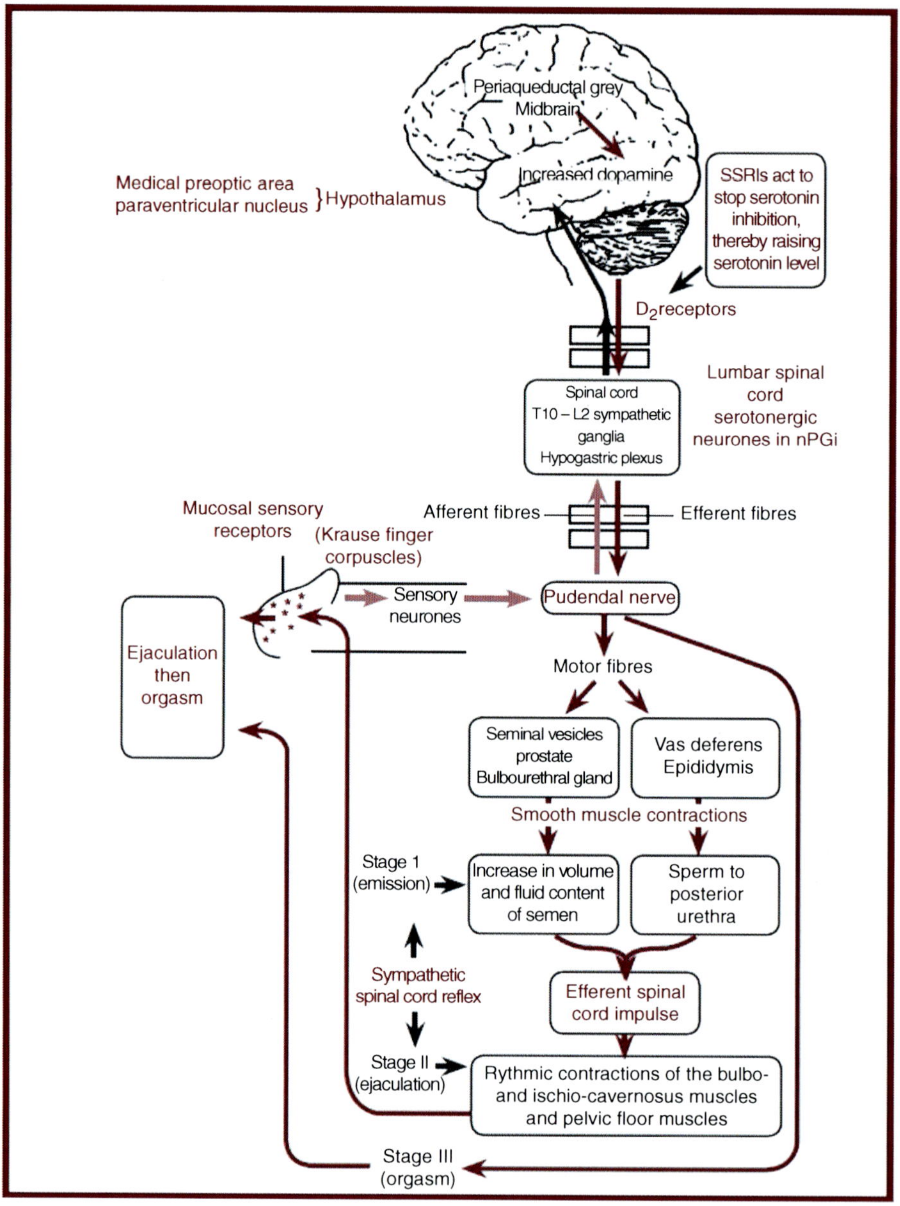

Fig. 16.1 Neural pathways for ejaculation (Reproduced with permission from Palmer and Stuckey (2008). © Copyright 2008)

- In the hypothalamus – 2 (the medial preoptic area and the paraventricular nucleus)
- In the midbrain – 1 (the periaqueductal gray)

These centers integrate the peripheral events of seminal emission, ejaculation, and orgasm. The efferent dopamine output by these centers is modulated by the nucleus paragigantocellularis. This has an inhibitory influence, from its serotonergic neurones in the brain and to the lumbar–sacral motor nuclei, which tonically inhibits ejaculation. Neurotransmitters involved in these centers include noradrenaline, γ-aminobutyric acid, oxytocin, nitric oxide, serotonin, and estrogen.

Ejaculation is triggered by efferent dopamine acting on the D2 receptors of central and spinal efferent fibers, which relay information down to the sympathetic ganglia at T10–L2 and sacral fibers. This stimulates pudendal nerve fibers from the S2–S4 region of the spinal cord, resulting in smooth muscle contractions of the prostate, seminal vesicles, vas deferens, and epididymis (*Stage I*).

Emission is a sympathetically mediated neural function (spinal nerves T10 through L2) that leads to contraction of the prostate gland and seminal vesicles, causing deposition of sperm/seminal fluid into the posterior urethra.

Expulsion is also a sympathetically mediated event (spinal nerves S2 through S4) that initiates with bladder neck closure and relaxation of the external striated urinary sphincter, causing rhythmic contraction of the skeletal pelvic floor muscles. The rhythmic contractions of the pelvic floor and bulbo- and ischiocavernosus muscles are controlled by parasympathetic nerves, which override sympathetic nerves. This propels seminal fluid out through the urethra, with resultant ejaculation (*Stage II*).

Orgasm is regarded as *Stage III*. Orgasm is the supremely pleasurable emotional and physical experience of climaxing, whereas by comparison, ejaculation, even though it is pleasurable, simply represents an unconscious reflex response that is generated by the effective and sexually prolonged stimulation of certain nerves in the genital region. Orgasm has more associations with the brain than with events in the pelvis, as is demonstrated, for example, by the fact that orgasm occurs during sleep.

Some men have been able to separate and recognize the different parts of the two processes of orgasm and ejaculation, which, on the one side, has let them experience multiple orgasms without having any ejaculation. On the other side, men may experience ejaculations with limited feelings of orgasmic pleasure. This information has bearing on the subject of premature ejaculation since premature ejaculation is usually not associated with the sexual fulfillment of an orgasm.

Primary premature ejaculation is possibly due to hyposensitivity of 5-hydroxytryptamine 2c (5-HT2c) serotonin receptors or hypersensitivity of 5-HT1 serotonin receptors, causing lowering of the ejaculatory threshold and shortened intravaginal ejaculatory latency time.

Theories of the Etiology of Premature Ejaculation

Theories of the etiology of premature ejaculation have focused on both *neurophysiologic* and *behavioral* components (Patrick et al. 2007; Semans 1956; Wolpe and Lazarus 1968). Until recently, premature ejaculation was believed to be predominantly a psychological disorder. Many researchers now believe that primary premature ejaculation is caused mostly by neurophysiologic factors, while secondary premature ejaculation may have mainly psychological contributors.

Somatic theories of premature ejaculation include penile hypersensitivity (reaching ejaculatory threshold more rapidly and/or having a lower ejaculatory threshold), a hyperexcitable ejaculatory reflex (faster emission/expulsion phase, faster bulbocavernosus reflex, or both), genetic predisposition (there may be a higher incidence of premature ejaculation in men whose first-degree relatives have premature ejaculation) and, as outlined above, central 5-HT receptor sensitivity (possible lower 5-HT neurotransmission, 5-HT2c receptor hyposensitivity and/or 5-HT1a receptor hypersensitivity, as suggested in animal models).

Also behavioral theories of premature ejaculation have been proposed which view premature ejaculations as learned behavior conditioned from early sexual experiences (Patrick et al. 2007; Semans 1956; Wolpe and Lazarus 1968). Poor sexual education, masturbation guilt, limited sexual privacy, and religious or cultural inhibitions have been proposed as precipitating factors. Therefore, in more recent years, sex therapists have focused more on the role of anxiety in the disorder. They suggest that anxiety may distract from the premonitory sensations that precede ejaculation and activate the sympathetic nervous system or lower the ejaculatory threshold. Additionally, these men may not be able to monitor and adequately manage their bodies' response to the sensations of escalating levels of sexual arousal. In all likelihood premature ejaculation may not have a single etiology but rather consists of multiple variable subtypes caused by varying contributing factors of biological and psychological origin.

Etiology of Secondary Premature Ejaculation

The most common cause of secondary premature ejaculation is a decline in erectile function. Epidemiologic studies have found a high rate of correlation between premature ejaculation and erectile dysfunction. In one large study, 41 % of men who reported erectile dysfunction also reported premature ejaculation, and 30 % of men reporting premature ejaculation also had erectile dysfunction. Other studies confirm this observation. The explanation advanced for the association between secondary premature ejaculation and declining erectile function is that rapid ejaculation becomes a compensatory mechanism, either conscious or unconscious, for the inability to maintain the erection. An alternative explanation is that lower levels of nitric oxide and increased sympathetic tone, associated with ageing, both predispose to erectile failure and hasten ejaculation. Although erectile dysfunction increases strongly in prevalence with age, premature ejaculation does not.

Approach to Treatment

Treating secondary PE should be within the scope of most GP's unlike primary PE which often requires skilled mental healthcare expertise (Waldinger et al. 2007; Assalian 2005). The approach to treating secondary or acquired premature ejaculation is to treat the underlying condition. Practice "the art of medicine" and reassure the patient he is anatomically normal. Check for signs and symptoms of chronic systemic disease, endocrine dysfunction, or gynecomastia. Also check gait, muscle strength, the sacral reflex arc, S2–S4 and general reflexes. It is important to perform a general medical examination as well as a genital examination.

Investigations are rarely needed in a younger patient with lifelong premature ejaculation. In older men with acquired premature ejaculation, especially if secondary to erectile dysfunction, relevant risk factors, cardiovascular disease, hypertension, hyperlipidaemia, diabetes, obesity, obstructive sleep apnoea, Peyronie's disease, lower urinary tract symptoms, and hyperthyroidism, may be identified.

PE5 inhibitors (like sildenafil, tadalafil, and vardenafil) may be effective in treating erectile dysfunction but do not prevent detumescence once ejaculation has occurred (McMahon et al. 2005; Chen et al. 2003). By contrast, intracavernosal injections prolong an erection beyond the point of ejaculation. However, they are not recommended for treating primary premature ejaculation without coexisting erectile dysfunction, largely because of the lack of evidence for their use, but also because of the risk of priapism (especially in men without vascular compromise) and the risk of penile fibrosis with long-term use.

References

Assalian P. Guidelines for the pharmacotherapy of premature ejaculation. World J Urol. 2005;23:127–9.

Chen J, Mabjeesh NJ, Matzkin H, Greenstein A. Efficacy of sildenafil as adjuvant therapy to selective serotonin reuptake inhibitor in alleviating premature ejaculation. Urology. 2003;61:197–200.

International Society for Sexual Medicine. ISSM definition of premature ejaculation. http://www.issm.info/prod/system/main/index.asp. Accessed Mar 2008.

Kimura Y, Miyamoto A, Urano S, et al. The spinal monoaminergic systems relating to ejaculation. I. Ejaculation and dopamine. Andrologia. 1982;14:341–6.

McMahon CG, Stuckey BG, Andersen M, et al. Efficacy of sildenafil citrate (Viagra) in men with premature ejaculation. J Sex Med. 2005;2:368–75.

Palmer NR, Stuckey BGA. Premature ejaculation: a clinical update. Med J Aust. 2008;188(11):662–6.

Patrick DL, Rowland D, Rothman M. Interrelationships among measures of premature ejaculation: the central role of perceived control. J Sex Med. 2007;4:780–8.

Rosen RC. Prevalence and risk factors of sexual dysfunction in men and women. Curr Psychiatry Rep. 2000;2:189–95.

Semans JH. Premature ejaculation: a new approach. South Med J. 1956;49:353–8.

Sharlip ID. Guidelines for the diagnosis and management of premature ejaculation. J Sex Med. 2006;3 Suppl 4:309–17.

Waldinger MD. The neurobiological approach to premature ejaculation. J Urol. 2002;168: 2359–67.

Waldinger MD. Premature ejaculation: state of the art. Urol Clin North Am. 2007;34:591–9.

Waldinger MD, Olivier B. Selective serotonin reuptake inhibitor-induced sexual dysfunction: clinical and research considerations. Int Clin Psychopharmacol. 1998;13 Suppl 6:S27–33.

Waldinger MD, Zwinderman AH, Olivier B, Schweitzer DH. The majority of men with lifelong premature ejaculation prefer daily drug treatment: an observation study in a consecutive group of Dutch men. J Sex Med. 2007;4:1028–37.

Wolpe J, Lazarus AA. Behavior therapy techniques: a guide to the therapy of neuroses. New York: Pergamon; 1968.

Chapter 17
Initial Workup and Use of Assessment Tools

Ng Kok Kit

Introduction

In the past, it was thought that premature ejaculation is mainly psychogenic in nature. In fact, when premature ejaculation is part of the symptoms of erectile dysfunction, it has been inferred that the etiology of erectile dysfunction is more likely to be psychogenic in nature. However, with improving knowledge of the male sexual physiology, it is believed now that premature ejaculation has an organic basis (e.g., penile hypersensitivity and serotonin receptor dysfunction) rather than being just indicative of the patient's anxious state in approaching sexual intercourse.

It now remains to define premature ejaculation. The Second International Consultation on Sexual and Erectile Dysfunction defines PE as "ejaculation with minimal stimulation and earlier than desired before or soon after penetration, which causes bother or distress, and over which the sufferer has little or no voluntary control" (McMahon et al. 2004). The International Society for Sexual Medicine has defined *lifelong PE* as "Premature ejaculation is a male sexual dysfunction characterized by ejaculation which always or nearly always occurs prior to or within about 1 min of vaginal penetration; and inability to delay ejaculation on all or nearly all vaginal penetrations; and negative personal consequences, such as distress, bother, frustration and/or the avoidance of sexual intimacy" (McMahon et al. 2008).

The common themes in these definitions include:

- The time to ejaculation
- Inability to control or delay ejaculation
- Negative consequences like bother or distress from PE

Ng.K. Kit, MBBS (Singapore), FRCS (Glas), FRCS (Edin), FAMS (Urology)
Department of Urology, Changi General Hospital,
Singapore, Singapore

Andropause and Men's Health Clinic, Changi General Hospital,
Singapore, Singapore
e-mail: kok_kit_ng@cgh.com.sg

P.H.C. Lim (ed.), *Men's Health*,
DOI 10.1007/978-1-4471-4766-4_17, © Springer-Verlag London 2013

History

Premature ejaculation can be divided into *lifelong* (*primary*) or *acquired* (*secondary*) (Hatzimouratidis et al. 2010). Lifelong PE is characterized by onset from the first sexual experience and remains a problem throughout life. For lifelong PE, ejaculation can happen very fast, before vaginal penetration or very shortly after. For patients with acquired PE, they have normal ejaculation prior to the onset of the problem. Time to ejaculation is short but is not usually as fast as in lifelong PE.

PE should also be classified as being *situational* (under specific circumstances or with a specific partner) or *consistent*.

Time to ejaculation and degrees of sexual stimulation should also be noted.

Besides establishing the nature of PE, it is important to find out how his PE affects his sexual life.

Physical Examination

In most men with premature ejaculation, physical examination is likely to be normal. However, a complete physical examination may be useful to screen for other sexual dysfunction. This includes a rough endocrinological, neurological, and vascular examination and the examination of the external genitalia.

For endocrinological examination, virility can be assessed to look for signs of hypogonadism. For neurological examination, lower limb strength and reflexes, including planter and anal reflexes, should be assessed. Lower limb vascularity should be examined to look for signs of vascular disease.

For the external genitalia, the glans should be examined for any deformities. The examiner should also palpate the shaft of the penis to feel for plaques which is suggestive of Peyronie's disease. The testes should also be felt for the presence of nodules and size.

Investigations

Laboratory investigations are generally not necessary for assessment of PE. Specific investigations can be ordered on findings from history or physical examination, for example, endocrinopathies.

Instruments

How do we quantify objectively premature ejaculation? From the term itself, we know that ejaculation occurs prematurely. However, what do we mean by "premature?" Does it mean that ejaculation occurs before entry into the vagina? Or does it mean that it occurs shortly after entry? Or could it even mean that ejaculation occurs before when a man feels that it *ought* to be?

To help diagnose as well as monitor therapy for PE, clinicians and scientists have formulated various instruments. Intravaginal ejaculatory latency time (IELT) has been used for a long time but may be cumbersome for clinicians to use. Premature Ejaculation Diagnostic Tool (PEDT) is a more recent instrument, which could be more convenient as it involves the use of a self-administered questionnaire. Other instruments include Premature Ejaculation Profile (PEP) (Patrick et al. 2005), the Index of Premature Ejaculation (IPE), and the Male Sexual Health Questionnaire Ejaculatory Dysfunction (MSHQ-EjD) (Rosen et al. 2007).

IELT

IELT, or intravaginal ejaculatory latency time, refers to the time between penetration into the vagina and ejaculation. Ideally, it should be timed with a stop watch. As it takes two persons to perform sexual intercourse, the timing can be done by the man or his partner. Certain studies have shown that IELT timed by the partner tend to be shorter than that done by the man himself, sometimes by as much as half.

In everyday clinical practice, self-estimated IELT is sufficient.

The value of IELT by which PE is diagnosed has not been agreed upon, as there is significant overlap of IELT between men with and men without PE. Most studies use IELT of 1 or 2 min for the diagnosis of PE, but Waldinger (Waldinger et al. 2004) found that some studies use an IELT of as high as 5 min.

Going back to the definitions of PE, IELT reflects only time, which is only one of the three components in the statements. The other two aspects – of the inability to control and negative impact on quality of life – are equally important.

PEDT

PEDT, or Premature Ejaculation Diagnostic Tool, is a new tool to help clinicians to screen and assess PE and its treatment (Fig. 17.1).

PEDT uses a self-administered questionnaire. All respondents were asked five questions about ejaculation. Each question has five possible answers, with a number (0–4) assigned to each answer (Fig. 17.2).

A PEDT score is obtained by adding the total numbers of these five questions.

- PEDT score ≥ 11: Has PE
- PEDT score = 9 or 10: Probable PE
- PEDT score ≤ 8: No PE

The use of PEDT has been validated in a study by Symonds (Symonds et al. 2007).

This is a questionnarie to help identify men who may have problem with ejaculation too soon during sexual activity. Even if you do not have difficulties, please answer all the question.

- ► Please mark ✓the box that best represents your answer for each of the questions below.
- ► Please mark only one box each question.
- ► Remember there are no right or wrong answer to these questions.
- ► While your experiences may change from time to time , what we're interested in here is your general experience with intercourse.

Fig. 17.1 Instructions for filling up PEDT questionnaire

Definition

Ejaculation here refers ejaculation (relase of semen) after penetration (when your penis enters your partner)

	Not difficult at all	Somewhat difficult	Moderately difficult	Very difficult	Extremely difficult
1.How difficult is it you to delay ejaculation?	□0	□1	□2	□3	□4

	Almost never or never 0 %	Loss than half the time 25 %	About half the time 50 %	More than half the time 75 %	Almost always or always 100 %
2.Do you ejaculate before you want to?	□0	□1	□2	□3	□4
3.Do you ejaculate with very little stimulation?	□0	□1	□2	□3	□4

	Not at all	Slitghtly	Moderately	Very	Extremely
4.Do you feel frustrated because of ejaculating before you want to?	□0	□1	□2	□0	□4
5. How concerned are you that your time to ejaculation leaves your partner sexually unfulfilled?	□0	□1	□2	□3	□4

A PEDT score is obtained by adding the total numbers of these five questions

- PEDT score ≥ 11: Has PE
- PEDT score = 9 or 10 : Probable PE
- PEDT score ≤ 8 : No PE

The use of PEDT has been validated in study by Symonds

Fig. 17.2 PEDT score questionnaire

Conclusions

PE is defined more than just by the time. It also includes the inability to control or delay ejaculation, and it has negative consequences to quality of life. The diagnosis of PE can be gleaned from history alone. However, a general physical examination may help to detect other sexual dysfunction. Many trials on PE use IELT. Another instrument, PDET, is a self-administered questionnaire that might be useful for the assessment and monitoring of the therapy of PE.

References

Hatzimouratidis K, Amar E, Eardley I, et al. Guidelines on male sexual dysfunction: erectile dysfunction and premature ejaculation. Eur Urol. 2010;57:804–14.

McMahon CG, Abdo C, Incrocci L, et al. Disorders of orgasm and ejaculation in men. J Sex Med. 2004;1:58–65.

McMahon CG, Althof SE, Waldinger MD, et al. An evidence-based definition of lifelong premature ejaculation: report of the International Society for Sexual Medicine (ISSM) ad hoc committee for the definition of premature ejaculation. J Sex Med. 2008;5:1590–606.

Patrick DL, Althof SE, Pryor JL, et al. Premature ejaculation: an observational study of men and their partners. J Sex Med. 2005;2:358–67.

Rosen RC, Catania JA, Althof SE, et al. Development and validation of four-item version of Male Sexual health Questionnaire to assess ejaculatory dysfunction. Urology. 2007;69:805–9.

Symonds T, Perelman MA, Althof S, et al. Development and validation of a premature ejaculation diagnostic tool. Eur Urol. 2007;52:565–73.

Waldinger MD, Zwinderman AH, Schweitzer DH, et al. Relevance of methodological design for the interpretation of efficacy of drug treatment of premature ejaculation: a systematic review and meta-analysis. Int J Import Res. 2004;1:1–13.

Chapter 18
Initial Management of the Newly Diagnosed PE

Peter Huat Chye Lim

Introduction

The initial management of the patient with PE can be conveniently done by first dividing the condition as to whether it is primary or secondary PE. Decision making regarding management strategy follows and is heavily predicated on what is derived from an initial detailed history taking leading on to a stepwise management plan according to the algorithm shown in Fig. 18.1.

History

The history should determine whether premature ejaculation is lifelong (i.e., primary) or acquired (i.e., secondary) and assess the severity of the problem.

For completeness, screen for other medical conditions that might be relevant. For example, if the patient has angina with subsequent fear of myocardial infarction (MI) during sexual activity, he might present with PE when the actual underlying problem is his cardiac disease and his worry regarding MI. Resolution of the heart problem usually solves the PE.

P.H.C. Lim, MBBS, MMed(Surg), M.Inst.Urol(Lon) FAMS, D.Urol(Lon), FICS
Department of Andrology, Urology Continence Center, Gleneagles Hospital, Singapore, Singapore

H.T. Naval Medical School, Surabaya, Indonesia

Edith Cowan University, Joondalup, WA, Australia

Society for Men's Health Singapore, Midview City, Singapore

Gleneagles Medical Centre, Singapore, Singapore

Department of Urology, Changi General Hospital, Singapore, Singapore
e-mail: profpeter.lim@gmail.com

P.H.C. Lim (ed.), *Men's Health*,
DOI 10.1007/978-1-4471-4766-4_18,

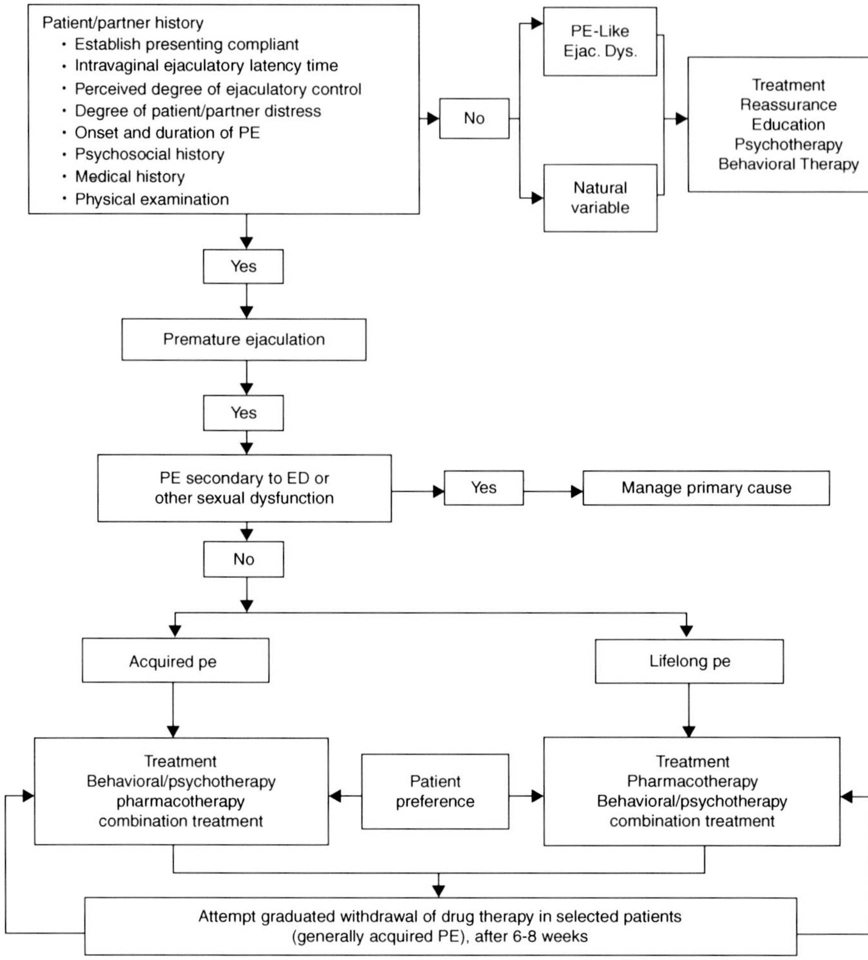

Fig. 18.1 Algorithm for the management of premature ejaculation (PE) (With permission of D. Rowland. Masters and Johnson (1970))

If the patient has always had PE from the time he began coitus, then he has primary PE. If he had successful coitus in the past and developed PE with the current relationship, then he has secondary premature ejaculation. In most cases, secondary PE is easier to treat and has a better prognosis.

- *Primary Premature Ejaculation* (Benson et al.)
  - *Prior psychological difficulties*, as psychiatric conditions, are more common in males with primary PE in the general population.
  - *Patient's early sexual experiences*. Any traumatic sexual episode as a child or teenager? For example, parental discovery of masturbation, with guilt feelings or punishment/threats for masturbation.

- *Family relationships* while growing up. What was the relationship with mother, father, brother(s), and sister(s)? Any history of incest or sexual assault? Males can be sexually assaulted by other males and, in rare instances, by females, including siblings.
- *Peer relationships* – male friends, female friends? *Self-regard* with respect to peers (e.g., inferior, superior, athletic, frail, more intelligent, less intelligent)?
- *Difficulties at work* (or school, if still a student)?
- General *attitude toward sex* (i.e., regarded as dirty), and what is the patient's sexual preference, fantasy, and arousal pattern?
- Strict *religious upbringing*? If so, what was he taught about sex?
- *Guilt feelings* when PE began with earlier nonmarital relationship.
- If PE started from first coital marital relationship, ask about *premarital, non-coital sexual play* between the partners.
- Sexual attitude and *response of the female partner*; any dyspareunia which could relate to the male's problem or may have preceded it.
- *Nonsexual part of the relationship* – fights, power struggles?
- If sexual partner is not present, ask why (i.e., *partner not supportive* or blaming him).
- Clues from these and similar questions usually point toward causation factors.

• *Secondary Premature Ejaculation* (Benson et al.)

- Prior relationships when PE was not present and any prior relationships in which transient episodes of PE occurred.
- In the current relationship, *was PE always a problem*, or did it start after an initial time frame when coitus was OK to both partners?
- Quality of the relationship vis-a-vis *nonsexual factors*. Partners get along mostly or conflict present? Who is dominant, and is the relationship equal?
- If *female sexual partner who accompanies him* did not come with him, ask why. She may regard the problem as only his rather than a couple issue.
- Does he have *impotence*? If he has erectile dysfunction (ED), did it begin after the PE or before? If no ED, what is the general timing for PE for the male – intromission, or what stage later?
- Was actual *coitus achieved or prevented by PE*?
- Is PE present at self-stimulation (i.e., masturbation), with nonintercourse stimulation by the partner, or *just with coitus*?
- *Time required for the female partner to reach climax*. Climax with intercourse, or requires direct clitoral stimulation (oral or manual) to be able to climax?
- If *ED began after the PE*, then treatment of both conditions may be required; ED may resolve when confidence in controlling ejaculation is restored. If ED started initially, PE may be a secondary sexual dysfunction, which resolves upon successful treatment of ED.

Physical Examination

Usually, the physical examination is normal in males whose only presenting condition is premature ejaculation. However, chronic preputial infection or inflammation/balanitis or an uncorrected phimosis may be found, and correction of the latter may help resolve PE. Abnormal penile curvatures and thin and atrophic skin of the prepuce and glans penis can contribute to the condition if left unresolved.

Causes of Premature Ejaculation

The cause of premature ejaculation is usually considered psychological in the main although this has not been definitively confirmed. Recent reports (Guiliano, 2010, Spinal reflex centre for ejaculation, personal communication) have located the ejaculatory center in the lower lumbar spinal cord, and disorders of this center may be causative.

- Primary Premature Ejaculation
  - In *primary PE and no prior sexual experiences, a deep-seated emotional disturbance* may be present, and the causes may be multiple.
  - Behavior may be a *conditioned response* resulting from teen masturbatory practice, or there is *deep anxiety* about sex connected to past traumatic experiences, e.g., family incest, sexual assault, and conflict with one or both parents.
  - *Consultation* with a psychiatrist and psychologist may be needed.
- Secondary Premature Ejaculation
  - Some type of *performance anxiety* is often present.
  - Performance pressure (i.e., fear of failure to satisfy the partner) can arise from *various precipitating events*, e.g., *ED*.
  - Careful history is needed because the situation may be *complex*.
  - If ED is not the problem, the *partner may have difficulty achieving climax* through intercourse and may require direct clitoral stimulation to reach a climax. And this is not communicated to him.
  - Most doctors are not trained sex therapists; *sorting out conflicts* in the relationship may need referral if simple counseling and/or medication is unsuccessful.

Differential Diagnoses and Other Problems (Benson et al.)

- In anorgasmia, or severely delayed orgasm in the female partner, nearly all men would be considered to have PE.
- Adverse effect from a psychotropic drug: If PE occurred after starting the drug but ceases when the drug is withdrawn.

- Pre-ejaculate: This may be confused as PE. Pre-ejaculate is the lubricating fluid produced by Cowper glands and other glands during the excitement phase of sexual stimulation. Reassurance of the male is needed.
- Erectile dysfunction (ED): This may occur in some men who are actually having premature ejaculation. Differentiating between the two problems is important.

Workup and Laboratory Studies (Benson et al.)

- In males with PE and no other medical problems, no specific lab tests aid or affect treatment.
- Checking serum testosterone (free, total, or bioavailable) level and prolactin level is useful if PE presents together with impotence.
- If depression or other conditions coexist, lab studies specific to depression or to other medical or psychological problems are appropriate.
- Occasionally vibrational threshold testing or nerve conduction time, somatosensory latency testing, or both are useful in a research setting.

Medical Care

Medical treatment for PE includes several options and must also include treatment of any concomitant erection problem. Include the female partner as much as possible in the treatment and counseling sessions in order to achieve the optimal response.

Treatment of Premature Ejaculation

The principles of therapy are essentially:
- Lifelong PE – pharmacotherapy.
- Acquired or situational PE – pharmacotherapy and/or behavioral therapy in particular men with significant contributing psychogenic or relationship factors may benefit from concomitant behavioral therapy.

Counseling/Behavioral Therapy

- Stop/start
- Squeeze technique
- Postcoital masturbation
- Sensate focus relationship counseling (best done by trained professional)

Withdrawal of Pharmacotherapy

- Attempt gradual withdrawal of drugs once condition stabilizes.

Behavioral Therapy: Strategy (Benson et al.)

Performance Anxiety

Treat performance anxiety/relieve underlying performance pressure on the male.

- If PE occurs at intercourse, the couple should be instructed that intercourse should not be attempted until PE is treated. The male may use manual stimulation, oral sex, or other means to satisfy the female partner meantime.
- If the male always experiences ejaculation with initial sexual excitement or early foreplay, this probably indicates primary PE.

Sexual Therapy

Treat couple with the stop-start or squeeze-pause technique (Masters and Johnson 1970)

The "stop-start" method:

- This technique involves sexually stimulating the man until he feels like he is about to reach orgasm. Stop the stimulation for about 30 s and then start it again. Repeat this pattern until the man wants to ejaculate. The last time continue stimulation until the man reaches orgasm.

The "squeeze" method: (Masters and Johnson 1970)

- This technique involves sexually stimulating the man until he recognizes that he is about to ejaculate. At that point, the man or his partner gently squeezes the end of the penis (where the glans meets the shaft) for several seconds. Stop sexual stimulation for about 30 s, and then, start it again. The person or couple may repeat this pattern until the man wants to ejaculate. The last time continue stimulation until the man reaches orgasm.

Precoital Masturbation

If the male is relatively young and can achieve another erection in a few minutes following an episode of premature ejaculation, he may find that his control is much better the second time.

- Advise young men to masturbate (or have their partner stimulate them rapidly to climax) 1–2 h before sexual relations are planned.
- The interval for achieving a second climax often includes a much longer period of latency, and the male can usually exert better control in this setting.
- In an older man, such a strategy may be less effective because the older man may have difficulty achieving a second erection after his first rapid sexual release. If this occurs, it can damage his confidence and may result in secondary impotence (Fig. 24.5).

Pharmacological Treatment of PE

- Selective serotonin reuptake inhibitors (SSRIs)
- PDE-5 inhibitors
- Topical local anesthetics

NB: For SSRIs, only Dapoxetine has regulatory approval for treatment of PE.

The most effective pharmacologic modality found to aid men with premature ejaculation is the selective serotonin reuptake inhibitors (SSRIs) class, drugs which are used normally as antidepressants in the clinical setting.

- Some tricyclic antidepressants with SSRI-like activity yield the same result.
- As a side effect, many of these agents have been found to cause a significant delay in reaching orgasm in both male and female patients.
- For this reason, medications with SSRI side effects have been used in men who experience premature ejaculation.

Medical Therapy Options for the Treatment of Premature Ejaculation (Fig. 24.2)

Nonselective serotonin reuptake inhibitors:

- Clomipramine
- Anafranil 25–50 mg/day or 25 mg 4–24 h pre-intercourse

Selective serotonin reuptake inhibitors:

- Anafranil, Fluxetine(Prozac)(Sarafern), Paroxetine(Paxil)
- Sertraline(Zoloft): 5–20 mg/day, 10, 20, 40 mg/day, or 20 mg, or 3–4 h pre-intercourse, 25–200 mg/day or 50 mg 4–8 h pre-intercourse

Dapoxetine (Pryor et al. 2006; Safarinejad 2006, 2008) (Fig. 24.4)

Dapoxetine is an SSRI developed specifically for the treatment of premature ejaculation. Dapoxetine is an approved SSRI for PE in seven European Union countries, including Sweden, Austria, Italy, New Zealand, and South Korea. It is rapidly absorbed (Tmax-1.5 h) following oral administration. It acts by decreasing brain concentrations of 5HT metabolites (5-HIAA). Dapoxetine may be effective at first dose (i.e., on-demand) for premature ejaculation when given 1–3 h prior to sexual intercourse, with an adverse-effect profile comparable to those of other SSRIs. Dapoxetine is under review for approval in Singapore and will be available for use soon.

Topical Therapies

- Lidocaine 2.5 % cream
- EMLA cream
- Prilocaine 2.5 % 20–30 min pre-intercourse

  Use of desensitizing creams for the male:

- In Korea and other areas of the Far East, SS cream (a combination of nine ingredients, mainly herbal; SS stands for Super Secret) has been shown to desensitize the penis, decrease the vibratory threshold, and help men with premature ejaculation to significantly delay their ejaculatory response (Choi et al. 2000; Xin et al. 1995).
- Unfortunately, SS cream is not yet approved by the US Food and Drug Administration (FDA), but simple combinations of lidocaine cream or related topical anesthetic agents can be used with similar effects, and they are safe as long as the patient has no history of allergy to the substance (Busato and Galindo 2004; Henry and Morales 2003).

PDE 5 Inhibitors in the Treatment of PE

- Can be used in older patients with PE or in those who have concomitant ED.
- PDE5 inhibitors can be employed alone or in combination with SSRIs when SSRIs alone fail to treat PE.
- Behavioral therapy should be used to prevent the recurrence of PE following withdrawal of PDE5-Is.
- For the PE patient with a definite etiological cause, the etiology should be cured first; if PE still exists, then PDE5-Is should be prescribed.

Concomitant ED and PE

ED and PE frequently overlap. When both are present, *erectile dysfunction should be treated first.* In the PE patient with a definite etiological cause, the etiology should be cured first.

The choice of therapeutic approach should:

- PDE-5 inhibitors
- PDE-5 inhibitors + SSRIs or *topical anesthetics*
- Pharmaceuticals + sex therapy (behavioral therapy) (Fig. 24.3)

Surgical Care

No recommended surgical treatment per se exists for premature ejaculation. However, chronic preputial infection or inflammation/balanitis or an uncorrected phimosis may occasionally be found, and correction of the latter may help resolve PE. Abnormal penile curvatures can contribute to the condition if left uncorrected. A urological opinion under these circumstances is mandated. Denervation techniques are still largely experimental and not currently deemed appropriate.

Consultations

- Consultation with a sex therapist, psychologist, or psychiatrist may prove helpful if the primary care physician or urologist cannot provide successful treatment or does not have the time to explore psychological issues and implement behavioral techniques (e.g., squeeze-pause). Some doctors are comfortable implementing medication therapy but not behavioral therapy. The patient should be offered all treatment options.
- For men who may be experiencing a severe emotional disturbance that is an underlying factor for PE, referral to a mental health professional is appropriate.

Prevention

- The incidence of PE in young men may possibly be decreased by better sex education during adolescence. Early successful treatment of ED in like fashion possibly prevents secondary PE in older men.

Complications

- Severe premature ejaculation can cause stress within a marriage or other relationships, which might contribute to conflicts and separation or divorce.
- Conception is also difficult in cases of premature ejaculation before vaginal intromission.

Prognosis

- Masters and Johnson state that the great majority of men with PE (>85 %) can be treated successfully with the squeeze-pause technique alone within 3 months of therapy. Others have observed much poorer success (Patrick et al. 2005).
- With a combination of methods including use of SSRI type medications, improvement or cure is possible provided that the couple (not just the man) is committed.
- Counseling and medical therapy can help achieve success rates as high as 85 %.
- The problem with all treatments for PE is that the relapse rate is 20–50 %. Hence, a long-term commitment to periodically repeating the behavioral techniques is needed. Some who succeed with medical therapy, i.e., SSRIs, may need to use the medication for the rest of their lives.

Patient Education

- Patients with premature ejaculation may be referred to a sex therapist, psychologist, psychiatrist, or marital counselor for additional help.
- Numerous books and articles in the lay press are available.
- Many can also find information on the Internet regarding this subject.

References

American Psychiatric Association. Diagnostic and statistical manual of mental disorders. 4th ed. Washington, D.C.: APA Press; 1994.

Benson A, Ost LB, Noble MJ, Lakin M. Premature ejaculation: over view of presentation and treatment. http://emedicine.medscape.com/article/435884-overview. Accessed on 6 Dec 2012.

Busato W, Galindo CC. Topical anaesthetic use for treating premature ejaculation: a double-blind, randomized, placebo-controlled study. BJU Int. 2004;93(7):1018–21.

Choi HK, Jung GW, Moon KH, et al. Clinical study of SS-cream in patients with lifelong premature ejaculation. Urology. 2000;55(2):257–61.

Henry R, Morales A. Topical lidocaine-prilocaine spray for the treatment of premature ejaculation: a proof of concept study. Int J Impot Res. 2003;15(4):277–81.

Masters WH, Johnson VE. Premature ejaculation. In: Human sexual inadequacy. Boston: Little Brown & Company; 1970. p. 92–115.

Patrick DL, Althof SE, Pryor JL, Rosen R, Rowland DL, Ho KF, et al. Premature ejaculation: an observational study of men and their partners. J Sex Med. 2005;2(3):358–67.

Pryor JL, Althof SE, Steidle C, Rosen RC, Hellstrom WJ, Shabsigh R, et al. Efficacy and tolerability of dapoxetine in treatment of premature ejaculation: an integrated analysis of two double-blind, randomised controlled trials. Lancet. 2006;368(9539):929–37.

Safarinejad MR. Comparison of dapoxetine versus paroxetine in patients with premature ejaculation: a double-blind, placebo-controlled, fixed-dose, randomized study. Clin Neuropharmacol. 2006;29(5):243–52.

Safarinejad MR. Safety and efficacy of dapoxetine in the treatment of premature ejaculation: a double-blind, placebo-controlled, fixed-dose, randomized study. Neuropsychopharmacology. 2008;33(6):1259–65.

Xin ZC, Choi YD, Seong DH, Choi HK. Sensory evoked potential and effect of SS-cream in premature ejaculation. Yonsei Med J. 1995;36(5):397–401.

Chapter 19
Premature Ejaculation: Simple Behavioral Therapy Steps

Adrian Wang Chee Cheng

Introduction

There are many factors that may cause premature ejaculation (PE). For many men, the problem may be related to anxiety. Anxiety often sets up a chain of events that may worsen things. The more you worry about the problem, the worse it gets. Other factors that can cause PE are faulty learned behaviors – such as climaxing too quickly during masturbation; relationship conflict with one's partner, which leads to tension and stress; and feelings of guilt and inadequacy about sex that may cause one to rush through intercourse.

Behavioral Therapy Steps

Here are some simple steps to deal with PE:

1. *Exercise.*
   Being fit and healthy will boost your confidence. If you feel good about yourself physically, your confidence in bed will naturally improve. Specific pelvic muscle exercises are important, too. Learn to tighten and strengthen the pubococcygeus muscle. This is the muscle that controls urine flow and ejaculation. Isolate that muscle by stopping your urine flow the next time you go to the bathroom. That is the muscle you need to strengthen.
2. *Manage stress.*
   Learn to manage expectations of yourself and your relationship. If you are feeling tense and rushed all the time, it will affect your sexual performance. Yoga,

A.W.C. Cheng, MBBS (Singapore), MMed (Psychiatry), FAMS
Department of Psychiatry, Gleneagles Hospital Singapore, Gleneagles Medical Centre, Singapore, Singapore

Department of Psychological Medicine, National University of Singapore, Singapore, Singapore
e-mail: adrian@wangpsych.com

P.H.C. Lim (ed.), *Men's Health*,
DOI 10.1007/978-1-4471-4766-4_19, © Springer-Verlag London 2013

meditation, and slow, deep breathing exercises can help defuse stress. Spend a few moments everyday to lower your stress levels.

3. *Improve communication with your partner.*
   Talk about the issue in an open, nonconfrontational way. Be comfortable with each other, find out what arouses her in bed, and learn to feel calm and confident when you are naked together in bed.
4. *Learn to stop and start.*
   This technique involves masturbating alone. During the first few times, masturbate in private without lubrication. Once you are close to climaxing, immediately stop and let the feeling subside. Do this a few times until you are confident of controlling your orgasm. Next, you can try masturbating with lubrication. Again, try to build the sensations up to the point you feel are about to climax, and then, stop. The idea is to train yourself to get comfortable with increasing levels of arousal. Gradually, you will be able to last longer before reaching that point of no return.
5. *Practice the squeeze technique.*
   If you feel like you are about to climax during sexual activity with your partner, get her to apply gentle but firm pressure where the head of the penis joins the shaft. Continuing squeezing until the urge to ejaculate subsides. Wait for half a minute to a minute, then resume sexual activity. If the urge to ejaculate returns, reapply the squeeze technique again. This technique helps you get used to the feeling of controlling the urge to ejaculate, and with time, you will be able to delay reaching orgasm too quickly.
6. *Self-distraction.*
   This is like the stop-start and squeeze methods, except you control the urge to ejaculate but suddenly thinking of something nonsexual, such as football.
7. *Think positive.*
   Use positive imagery to enhance your bedroom confidence. Instead of focusing on failure, tell yourself you are a good lover, and that you will be able to please your partner. By focusing on positive feelings, you will distract yourself from feelings of stress.
8. *Find the right position.*
   Find a sexual position that you find relaxing and comfortable. Being on top may not necessarily be the best option because supporting your weight with your arms may increase overall muscle tension. Instead, try the female on top or side-to-side position Kaplan (1975–1987).

Try these behavioral techniques and figure out which one works best for you. Remember – practice is the key. Think positive and do not despair if things do not go well at first. PE is a very treatable condition.

Reference

Kaplan HS. The illustrated manual of sex therapy. 2nd ed. New York: Brunner-Routledge; 1975–1987.

Chapter 20
Choice of Pharmacologic Agents

P. Ganesan Adaikan and B. Srilatha

Historically, premature ejaculation (PE) was considered to be an acquired psychosexual phenomenon. Hence, behavioral therapies such as "stop-start" and "squeeze" methods were popular management approaches albeit with limited success. Observation of delayed ejaculation in patients taking selective serotoninergic reuptake inhibitors (SSRI) has contributed to the serendipitous advent of pharmacotherapy using SSRI for PE. Serotonin on the whole exerts an inhibitory effect on ejaculation both at the spinal and supraspinal levels. Many serotonin receptor subtypes have been identified so far, each having different functions. Other neurotransmitters implicated to play a secondary role in ejaculatory process include dopamine, acetylcholine, adrenaline, neuropeptides, oxytocin, gamma aminobutyric acid, and nitric oxide.

Current management approach for PE thus includes behavioral therapy which can be combined with daily or on-demand use of pharmacologic agents such as the SSRIs, topical/local anesthetics, opioid agonists, and PDE5 inhibitors. In recent times, the SSRIs, which are commonly used antidepressants, have been tried successfully to treat PE given the knowledge that delayed ejaculation is a common side effect of these drugs. As such, the SSRIs or tricyclic antidepressants including paroxetine, sertraline fluoxetine, citalopram, fluvoxamine, and clomipramine are able to prolong the objective index of intravaginal ejaculatory latency time (IELT) by several minutes. The SSRIs, as implied by the name, and the tricyclic antidepressants interfere with the reuptake of 5-HT from the synaptic clefts by the transporter mechanisms, with the resultant increase in serotonergic neurotransmission and activation of postsynaptic 5-HT2C receptors; this is expected to mediate the desired therapeutic effect of an ejaculatory delay.

P.G. Adaikan, Ph.D., D.Sc., ACS (✉) • B. Srilatha, M.D., Ph.D.
Department of Obstetrics and Gynaecology, Yong Loo Lin School of Medicine,
National University Hospital, National University of Singapore,
NUHS Tower Block Level 12, 1E Kent Ridge Road, Singapore 119228, Singapore
e-mail: p_ganesan_adaikan@nuhs.edu.sg

P.H.C. Lim (ed.), *Men's Health*,
DOI 10.1007/978-1-4471-4766-4_20, © Springer-Verlag London 2013

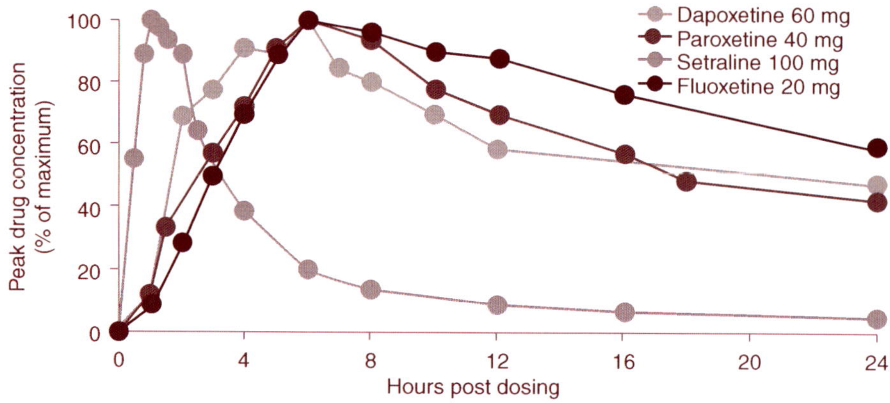

Fig. 20.1 Dapoxetine plasma concentrations at 24 h are <5 % of peak levels (Andersson et al. 2006)

Results from several studies have shown that a daily chronic dosing of SSRI significantly prolonged IELT in men with PE. In the relative order of efficacy, paroxetine (20 mg/day) was found to be superior to sertraline (50 mg/day), fluoxetine (20 mg/day), or citalopram (40 mg/day) with the mean IELT increase from baseline in the range of 1.5–7 min compared to placebo (Waldinger et al. 2004a; McMahon 2002) (Fig. 20.1). However, the usefulness of these drugs may be limited by other sexual effects such as diminished erectile function/libido and anorgasmia and other systemic side effects (GI manifestations, headache, lethargy, ataxia, anxiety, insomnia, etc.) (Hellstrom 2009). Also, in view of the possibility of an abrupt discontinuation syndrome marked by severe systemic manifestations, it is advisable to gradually taper the SSRI-dosing over several weeks while ending treatment (Sadeghi-Nejad and Watson 2008).

Along these lines, an "on-demand" use of SSRIs has been considered to be safer, with less propensity for the adverse effects of chronic dosing (Waldinger et al. 2004b). Furthermore, it may be more efficacious to combine it with a 5-HT$_{1A}$ receptor antagonist or other agents that accentuated the 5-HT release (Gurkan et al. 2008). Indeed, a short-acting SSRI, dapoxetine, which has been approved for use in several European countries as an "on-demand" medication for PE, has proven to be a potent inhibitor of the 5-HT transporter at the synaptic cleft of central and peripheral serotonergic neurons (Andersson et al. 2006). When used in doses of 30 or 60 mg, there is a rapid absorption with attainment of peak plasma levels in 1.01 and 1.27 h; there is also rapid elimination (1.3–1.4 h) with minimal accumulation in the body (Fig. 20.1) (Modi et al. 2006).

It has been documented that dapoxetine, in the recommended doses of 30 and 60 mg taken 30–60 min prior to an intercourse, significantly increased the IELT duration to 3.03 and 3.15 min compared to placebo (1.66 min). If the dosing occurred

3–4 h before, the IELT increased to 3.06 and 3.97 min, respectively, in comparison to placebo administration (1.79 min) (Pryor et al. 2006). Additionally, dapoxetine also improved other parameters of sexual satisfaction; it is moderately well tolerated with low-reported incidences of adverse effects, abrupt withdrawal events, and need for discontinuation.

Similar to SSRIs, the tricyclic antidepressant, clomipramine also significantly increased IELT both with continuous dosing and as an "on-demand" agent. With comparable pharmacokinetics as most SSRIs, the IELT increase to fourfold from baseline indicates its therapeutic efficacy; however, there may be higher incidences of side effects (Waldinger et al. 2004b).

Another orally effective agent for PE is the μ-opioid receptor analgesic tramadol, which functions as a combined reuptake inhibitor of 5-HT, norepinephrine, and GABA. In two of the clinical trials using 25 or 50 mg of tramadol, there was a significant increase in IELT to about 4–8 min compared to the placebo arm (Salem et al. 2008). However, its reported efficacy and usefulness in PE may be compromised by an abuse potential in the clinical setting.

Currently available pharmacotherapeutic agents for ED, viz., the phosphodiesterase type 5 inhibitors (PDE-5Is) sildenafil, vardenafil, and tadalafil, have been tried in combination with SSRIs, particularly in patients with a coexistent ED. Aside from their usefulness in this cohort, trials evaluating PDE-5Is as an independent management option for PE have drawn variable outcomes involving the IELT data. In the presence of an SSRI, sildenafil or tadalafil significantly improved IELT, well above the SSRI arm, and the combination was also better in terms of overall satisfaction (Salonia et al. 2002; Mattos et al. 2008). However, the higher incidence of side effects to the combination precludes a routine use of these drugs in PE per se.

Topical formulations – creams, gels, or sprays – containing local anesthetic agents such as lidocaine and prilocaine have been commonly used over the years as effective treatment options for PE. In small clinical trials, the IELT increased to two- to four-folds following topical application of the cream (2.5 %) or an aerosol spray (metered-dose delivery system containing 7.5 mg of lidocaine and 2.5 mg of prilocaine/spray) (Dinsmore et al. 2006; Dinsmore and Wyllie 2009). A combination of local anesthetic, dyclonine with PGE_1, was also tested in a small cohort for its usefulness in reducing the sensations in the glans area; further studies are required to confirm the safety and efficacy of this combination (Gurkan et al. 2008). A mixture of nine Korean herbs has been used as a topical cream (severance-secret (SS) cream) with purported local anesthetic and desensitizing effect on the penile shaft and glans. In a randomized clinical trial, the IELT significantly increased to 11 min compared to placebo (2.5 min) (Choi et al. 1999). As such, topical agents can be used as and when required and are devoid of severe systemic side effects of the classical oral preparations. However, together with penile desensitization, there may be vaginal transmission resulting in incidences of numbness and reduced pleasure response in the female partner, particularly with the local anesthetic drugs.

References

Andersson KE, Mulhall JP, Wyllie MG. Pharmacokinetic and pharmacodynamic features of dapoxetine, a novel drug for "on demand" treatment of premature ejaculation. BJU Int. 2006;97:311–5.

Choi HK, Xin ZC, Choi YD, Lee WH, Mah SY, Kim DK. Safety and efficacy study with various doses of SS-cream in patients with premature ejaculation in a double-blind, randomized, placebo controlled clinical study. Int J Impot Res. 1999;11(5):261–4.

Dinsmore WW, Wyllie MG. PSD502 improves ejaculatory latency, control and sexual satisfaction when applied topically 5 min before intercourse in men with premature ejaculation: results of a phase III, multicentre, double-blind, placebo controlled study. BJU Int. 2009;103:940–9.

Dinsmore WW, Hackett G, Goldmeier D, et al. Topical eutectic mixture for premature ejaculation (TEMPE): a novel aerosol-delivery form of lidocaine-prilocaine for treating premature ejaculation. BJU Int. 2006;99:369–75.

Gurkan L, Oommen M, Hellstrom WJG. Premature ejaculation: current and future treatments. Asian J Androl. 2008;10(1):102–9.

Hellstrom WJG. Emerging treatments for premature ejaculation: focus on dapoxetine. Neuropsychiatr Dis Treat. 2009;5:37–46.

Mattos RM, Marmo Lucon A, Srougi M. Tadalafil and fluoxetine in premature ejaculation: prospective, randomized, double-blind, placebo-controlled study. Urol Int. 2008;80(2):162–5.

McMahon CG. Long-term results of treatment of premature ejaculation with selective serotonin re-uptake inhibitors. Int J Impot Res. 2002;14:S19.

Modi NB, Dresser MJ, Simon M, Lin D, Desai D, Gupta S. Single and multiple dose pharmacokinetics of dapoxetine hydrochloride, a novel agent for the treatment of premature ejaculation. J Clin Pharmacol. 2006;46(3):301–9.

Pryor JL, Althof SE, Steidle C, et al. Efficacy and tolerability of dapoxetine in treatment of premature ejaculation: an integrated analysis of two double-blind, randomized-controlled trials. Lancet. 2006;368(9539):929–37.

Sadeghi-Nejad H, Watson W. Premature ejaculation: current medical treatment and new directions. J Sex Med. 2008;5:1037–50.

Salem EA, Wilson SK, Bissada NK, Delk JR, Hellstrom WJ, Cleves MA. Tramadol HCl has promise in an on-demand use to treat premature ejaculation. J Sex Med. 2008;5(1):188–93.

Salonia A, Maga T, Colombo R, et al. A prospective study comparing paroxetine alone versus paroxetine plus sildenafil in patients with premature ejaculation. J Urol. 2002;168(6):2486–9.

Waldinger MD, Zwinderman AH, Schweitzer DH, Olivier B. Relevance of methodological design for the interpretation of efficacy of drug treatment of premature ejaculation: a systematic review and meta-analysis. Int J Impot Res. 2004a;16:369–81.

Waldinger MD, Zwinderman AH, Olivier B. On-demand treatment of premature ejaculation with clomipramine and paroxetine: a randomized, double-blind fixed-dose study with stop-watch assessment. Eur Urol. 2004b;46:510–5.

Chapter 21
Premature Ejaculation: Treatment of the Difficult Case and Advanced Counseling Techniques and When to Refer

Ng Beng Yeong

When reading about the role of psychotherapy in premature ejaculation, it is pertinent to note the two different schools of thoughts. The first school would recommend the conventional view offered by sex therapists that psychotherapy can help a man delay his ejaculation. A more radical view is offered by neuropsychiatrist Waldinger – psychotherapy is only indicated in men or couples who cannot accept premature ejaculation (Waldinger 2005). In contrast to the classical psychological view, Waldinger (2005) has suggested that the purpose of psychodynamic or cognitive psychotherapy is not to learn how to delay ejaculation but has to be how to cope with premature ejaculation, for example, in cases where medication has no or inadequate effect (Waldinger 2005).

Interestingly, Polonsky (2000) identified four different patterns and presentations of PE (Polonsky 2000):

1. "Simple" PE. The individual appears to have identified a wish for better control and has demonstrated an ability to engage in relationships that reflect mutuality and reciprocity. Therapy is sought out individually to help with mastery.
2. "Simple" plus "relational." This represents a variant of the first type. The individual is in a relationship, and the partner participates in the treatment. The PE is usually the identified complaint, but the couple seeks help to better manage the control of ejaculation and to improve communication skills between them.
3. "Complicated." The men in this group have complicated psychological issues that affect profoundly their ability to manage relationships. In addition, they suffer with PE and are hampered in their ability to involve a partner in a collaborative way.

Ng.B. Yeong
Department of Psychiatry, Singapore General Hospital, Singapore, Singapore

Department of Psychiatry, Duke-NUS Graduate Medical School, Yong Loo Lin School of Medicine, National University of Singapore, Singapore, Singapore
e-mail: ng.beng.yeong@sgh.com.sg

P.H.C. Lim (ed.), *Men's Health*,
DOI 10.1007/978-1-4471-4766-4_21,

4. "Complicated" and "relational." These couples are a challenge to the skills and creativity of the therapist. They each have complicated psychological difficulties, usually have severe conflicts around intimacy, and have had difficulty in integrating their feelings about sex.

Contemporary treatment approaches include an integrating of individual and couple dynamics, cognitive, and behavioral approaches.

Tips for Counseling

1. Oftentimes, PE is a couple's problem. Nevertheless, many single young men who are not in a committed relationship may also seek treatment for PE. It is important to engage the single men in treatment so that they can gain mastery on their own, which will help restore their self-esteem and sexual confidence.
2. Check the couple's expectations. Zilbergeld (1992) has addressed the unrealistic expectations in some men in *The New Male Sexuality*, where he describes the attributes of the "perfect penis" – hard as steel, always ready, and able to last forever (Zilbergeld 1992). It is important to have realistic expectations – the lovemaking experience typically lasts 15–45 min, with 2–12 min involving intercourse itself. For both the contemporary clinician and couples coming to grips with sexual concerns, the most important first step is education about anatomy, physiology, and expectations.
3. Be prepared to manage the partner's anger. Zilbergeld (1995) has written about the role of the angry or hostile spouse in the treatment of sexual problems (Zilbergeld 1995). Anger is known to increase anxiety, which creates a barrier to becoming more competent sexually (Zilbergeld 1995). PE is not unique in the sexual dysfunctions in that anxiety invariably makes the situation worse. For change to take place, a level of safety, trust, and patient collaboration is desirable.
4. Consider relationship issues. Sexual heath and satisfaction are usually embedded in a relationship with a partner and involve elements of passion, intimacy, caring, commitment, and communication (Rowland 2007). One needs to understand the dynamics of the couple and how they express their wishes and desires – what is perceived and what is misperceived. It is important to note the "kitchen sink syndrome" where couple will hurl insults at each other and talk about each others' misbehaviors and grievances and not stay behind to resolve any of the problems. In marital therapy, it will be useful to get the couple to prioritize their issues and learn to focus on a problem at a time.
5. Get the couple to describe their sexual scripts and to describe in detail the activities that they do for foreplay and the actual intimacy and sexual intercourse. Equally helpful is to facilitate communication between the couple about sexual issues and give permission regarding an expanded repertoire of behaviors for greater sexual satisfaction (Rowland 2007).

6. Behavioral techniques commonly used in the treatment of PE include "stop-start" and "squeeze" techniques; these require commitment from the man and his partner. For individuals who could have learnt the techniques from the Internet, it may be useful to check if they are using the correct steps. The "stop-start" technique involves the man stimulating himself to the point just before ejaculation and then stopping. Once the sensations have subsided, he starts again. This can be repeated three times. The length of time before each stop gets gradually longer. The "squeeze" technique involves the partner (or man) using their fingers to squeeze the head (glans) of the penis to cause the erection (and ejaculation) to subside. As the man is able to delay his ejaculation in time, intercourse is gradually introduced. It is usually recommended that a man learning to control ejaculation progresses from masturbating with no lubricant, to masturbating with lubricant, to intercourse with his partner on top of him while he lies still (so that his penis acclimates to being inside her vagina), and to intercourse with him on top and moving (Ng 2005).
7. The couple can be encouraged to enjoy a second intercourse after one involving a short ejaculation latency, to take advantage of the decreased sexual arousal most men experience during the refractory period (Rowland 2007). Many younger men would masturbate before anticipation of sexual intercourse in an attempt to overcome PE.
8. The couple can be encouraged to vary their intercourse-related behaviors to attenuate the patient's level of sexual arousal for the purpose of keeping it below the level of ejaculation inevitability (Rowland 2007).
9. The couple could be encouraged to experiment with the partner (e.g., female) in superior or lateral positions because these typically provide men with a greater sense of ejaculatory control. Other suggestions include slowing down during intercourse, breathing deeply, and having shallow penile penetration (Rowland 2007).
10. Consider the use of sensate focus techniques. These techniques permit enjoyment of physical sensations without necessarily generating sexual arousal and de-emphasize the focus on intercourse and orgasm within the sexual relationship and may help reduce the man's performance anxiety. Sensate focus therapy or sex therapy was first described by Masters and Johnson. When starting treatment, the rationale of treatment is explained, sexual education is given, and a temporary ban in intercourse is suggested. The partners then follow a program of homework exercises, including mutual nongenital and genital pleasuring, communication exercises, and exercises aimed at reducing performance demand and the resulting anxiety (Wincze & Carey 2001). Performance anxiety, which operates through sympathetic pathways, may serve to prime the ejaculatory response prematurely. The downside of sex therapy is that some couple may find the steps mechanical and their sexual interest may be adversely affected.
11. Think of comorbid erectile dysfunction. Some men with PE try to gain control over their body by denying themselves sensations. What is more useful is to allow oneself to enjoy the different levels of arousal that one is capable of experiencing.

12. Think of hypoactive sexual desire disorder in the women. Low sexual desire could be a consequence of problematic functioning in other domains of sexuality, the partner relationship, or the physical and psychological condition of the female client or her partner.
13. Consider the use of combined treatments – medications with psychological interventions (Ng 2005). Proponents of psychotherapy like to quote the axiom "If you only take a pill, you gain no skill." As the man and his partner gain a greater sense of self-efficacy, reliance on medications can be reduced.
14. Consider the importance of cognitions. In cognitive-behavioral therapy, one uses thought records to capture the cognitions that accompany emotions, for example, those that are manifested during sexual activity. In therapy, cognitive restructuring techniques are used to help patients modify their negative cognitions so that these thoughts are replaced by neutral or positive ones. For instance, a patient who has PE in one out of three sexual encounters may feel like a total failure in bed. In therapy, he can learn to look at the problem from a different perspective, for example, that it occurs in one out of three encounters and that there are still positive aspects of the sexual encounters that he and his partner can enjoy.
15. Invest time on relapse prevention. At this juncture, it is not known whether relapse occurs because the behavioral techniques become less effective with continued use or because couples merely stop using them once the novelty has worn off. Deliberate strategies to prevent relapse involve (a) predicting the likelihood of occasional "setbacks" and preparing couples appropriately and (b) using increased spacing between sessions as progress is noted (McCarthy 1993).
16. PE can generate a great amount of distress for those who are affected. It is important for the clinician to empathize with the patient and not to offer premature reassurance or diminish the severity of it by superficial remarks. Minimizing the problem is not only unhelpful but may make the individual feel even more isolated and misunderstood.

When to Refer

1. When PE is complicated by many marital and relationship issues
2. When the person with PE fails to respond to medications treatment or simple behavioral interventions
3. When the person with PE has significant psychiatric comorbidity of anxiety or depression (Ng 2003)
4. When the doctor is not adequately trained in psychosexual medicine or is uncomfortable dealing with sexual issues

References

McCarthy BW. Relapse prevention strategies and techniques in sex therapy. J Sex Marital Ther. 1993;19:142–6.

Ng BY. Strategies for helping depressed men with sexual dysfunctions. Singapore Family Physicians. 2003;29(4):91.

Ng BY. Coming of age: an integrated approach to premature ejaculation. Singapore Family Physicians. 2005;31(2):42–5.

Polonsky DC. In: Leiblum SR, Rosen RC, editor. Asessment and treatment of male sexual dysfunction in primary care. Principles and practice of sex therapy. 3rd ed. New York: The Guilford Press; 2000. p. 305–32.

Rowland DL. Sexual health and problems. In: Grant JE, Potenza MN, editors. Textbook of men's mental health. Washington, D.C.: American Psychiatric Publishing; 2007. p. 171–203.

Waldinger MD. Male ejaculation and orgasmic disorders. In: Handbook of sexual dysfunction. Boca Raton: Taylor and Francis Group; 2005. p. 215–48.

Wincze JP, Carey MP. Sexual dysfunction: a guide for assessment and treatment. New York: The Guilford Press; 2001.

Zilbergeld B. The new male sexuality. New York: Bantam Books; 1992.

Zilbergeld B. The critical and demanding partner in sex therapy. In: Rosen RC, Leiblum SR, editors. Case studies in sex therapy. New York: Guilford Press; 1995. p. 311–30.

Chapter 22
Management of the Infertile Couple When the Male Partner Has Ejaculatory Dysfunction

P. Ganesan Adaikan and Yap Seng Chong

Fertility and Ejaculation

From time immemorial, man had always been entangled in the web of strong procreative instinct as the pillar of his existence in this planet. If he is unable to achieve an erection or ejaculate appropriately or if the desire is unduly compromised due to hormone upheavals, his fertility may suffer leading to serious implications on the quality of couple relationship. The sexual problems may be independent or interdependent with abnormalities in sperm parameters and fertility or sexual issues in the female partner. Indeed, difficulty in conceiving a child can arise because of the abnormality in man's reproductive system or the woman's or a combination of both. Male causes are in the region of about one-third of the total infertility. While the major or direct cause of male infertility is the result of insufficient amount or production of healthy spermatozoa, fertility can be compromised if the man suffering from premature ejaculation (PE) deposits the ejaculate outside the vagina/in the introitus or half way through the vagina in an incomplete penetration (the lower limit for male fertility is 20 million spermatozoa per milliliter). Furthermore, a lower amount of spermatozoa in migration to the fallopian tube will make the conception even more difficult The male physiological function of ejaculation comprises emission of semen into the prostatic urethra and expulsion of the ejaculate by coordinated contractions of muscles of the pelvic floor, lower extremities, and trunk. While ejaculatory dysfunction can be multifactorial leading to diminished sexual pleasure as well as fertility, cases of PE need to be evaluated for the severity; particularly whether ejaculation takes place before penetration of the vagina. Accordingly, one should treat premature ejaculation (see Chaps. 4, 5, and 6) and any

P.G. Adaikan, Ph.D., D.Sc., ACS
Y.S. Chong, MBBS, MRCOG, MMed(O&G), FAMS, M.D. (✉)
Department of Obstetrics and Gynaecology,
Yong Loo Lin School of Medicine, National University Hospital,
National University of Singapore, Singapore, Singapore
e-mail: yschong@nus.edu.sg

P.H.C. Lim (ed.), *Men's Health*,
DOI 10.1007/978-1-4471-4766-4_22,

Type of sexual dysfunction	no.	(%)
Erectile dysfunction	695	(67.1)
Premature ejaculation	240	(23.2)
Unconsummation	101	(9.7)
Total	1,036	(100)

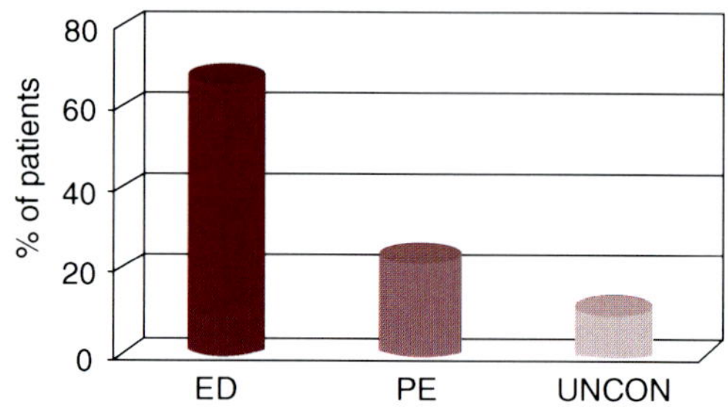

Fig. 22.1 Prevalence of unconsummation among SD patients (Adaikan et al. (2011))

other existing sexual dysfunction such as retrograde ejaculation (into the bladder) and erectile dysfunction, if any.

Premature Ejaculation

Premature ejaculation is also known as rapid ejaculation. It is the most common sexual problem in men, affecting 25–40 % of men (community prevalence). In our sexual dysfunction clinic, PE accounted for 23.2 % of male sexual dysfunction (MSD) cases seen (Fig. 22.1). While the incidence of unconsummated marriages is around 10 %, premature ejaculation was one of the direct causes of unconsummation and resultant infertility in these couples. According to Hassanzadeh and coworkers (2010), the prevalence of PE in infertile men can be as high as 43 %. When we studied the ethnic prevalence, 13.9 % of 424 Chinese MSD patients presented with non-consummation of their marriages; the incidence was 8.1 and 19.1 %, respectively, for 64 Malays and 146 Indians in this cohort. This shows that non-consummation of marriages was a major presentation for infertility at the OBGYN-andrology setting, National University Hospital (NUH).

Men with PE are known to suffer from bother, depression, and anxiety which can contribute to reduction of desire, libido, and frequency of attempts of intercourse and avoidance of intimacy due to embarrassments; this and resultant frustration of the wife can further compromise the chances of conception in a marital setting. The situation can also lead to emotionally and physically dissatisfied couple.

Delayed or Retarded Ejaculation

Delayed or retarded ejaculation is difficulty in achieving ejaculation despite the presence of adequate libido, sexual stimulation, and erectile capacity. When severe, the condition presents as ejaculatory incompetence with compromised fertility. Causes include marital disharmony and relationship issues, alcoholism and drug abuse, neurological and endocrine illnesses, diabetes, cancer, prostatic problems, and surgical trauma. High noradrenaline levels and sympathetic nervous system activation can block the arousal needed for orgasm.

Retrograde Ejaculation

During retrograde ejaculation, the seminal fluid is ejaculated backward into the urinary bladder. Patients with retrograde ejaculation usually achieve orgasm normally and give the history that the post-ejaculatory urine is cloudy. Diabetic neuropathy affects the autonomic nerve supply to the bladder neck, and about one-third of diabetics will have some degree of retrograde ejaculation. Other causes of retrograde ejaculation are spinal cord lesions and injuries, perineal surgeries, and several prescription drugs.

Pharmacological management has improved the clinical outcome to a certain extent in these patients. Sperm retrieval from the urinary bladder and assisted reproductive techniques has resolved the fertility concerns in the young couples.

Anejaculation

Anejaculation is characterized by the absence of ejaculation with well-preserved nocturnal penile tumescence and emissions. Treatment includes psychosexual counseling, drugs such as ephedrine and imipramine, and use of vibrator and electroejaculation (application of electrical current to stimulate ejaculation). Mechanical obstructions to the ejaculatory pathway, however, need surgical intervention.

Therapeutic Implications

In general, man derives satisfaction from giving pleasure to his partner, and meeting her expectation is very important to him. Therefore, when ejaculatory dysfunction strikes, the sufferer feels that he is letting his partner down and this thought can affect the quality of life with deep emotional impact and loss of self-esteem. In a stable relationship, this can create a downward spiral leading to withdrawal, isolation, and depression. The present-day treatment options and the awareness have brought back the feelings of intimacy in couple relationships. Together with specific treatment for the different type of ejaculatory dysfunction, it is imperative to address interpersonal issues and impress upon the need for lifestyle modifications and stress control for long-term successful outcomes in the context of both procreational and recreational sexuality.

References

Hassanzadeh K, Yavari-kia P, Ahmadi-Asrbadr Y, Nematzadeh-Pakdel A, Alikhah H. Features of premature ejaculation in infertile men. Pak J Biol Sci. 2010;13:911–5.

Adaikan PG, Linton DJ. Premature ejaculation and ED a comparison of the two most frequent sexual dysfunctions. J Sex Med. 2011;8(3):84–299.

Chapter 23
Delayed/Retarded Ejaculation

Louis Gooren

Definition

Delayed ejaculation, also called retarded ejaculation, is the difficulty in ejaculating, even with a firm erection and sufficient sexual arousal and stimulation.

Presentation

A man with the condition of retarded ejaculation simply cannot achieve orgasm, even if he has experienced what would seem to be normal levels of sexual excitement. This may happen all the time, or he may find that he is unable to attain orgasm in any circumstances, sometimes even during masturbation. The Diagnostic and Statistical Manual of Mental Disorders (DSM-IV-TR) puts this disorder among the sexual dysfunctions, along with rapid ejaculation.

Delayed ejaculation results in considerable distress, anxiety, and lack of sexual confidence for those suffering from it. Furthermore, men with partners often experience impairment of both the sexual and nonsexual aspects of their relationships, with such negative effects compounded when procreation is a consideration.

Like all sexual problems, delayed ejaculation occurs in all kinds of men, of all intelligence levels, professions, and ages. It may begin to develop around the time of puberty, or it may commence later in life.

L. Gooren, M.D., Ph.D.
Department of Endocrinology, Free University of Amsterdam, Amsterdam, the Netherlands

H.T. Naval Medical School, Surabaya, Indonesia
e-mail: louisjgooren@gmail.com

P.H.C. Lim (ed.), *Men's Health*,
DOI 10.1007/978-1-4471-4766-4_23,

Types

Retarded ejaculation is estimated to occur in 1–4 % of men. Delayed ejaculation can be classified as either primary or secondary. Primary delayed ejaculation is when a man has never been able to ejaculate during sexual intercourse. Secondary delayed ejaculation is when a man was able to ejaculate during intercourse at one time in his life but no longer is able to, or he does so infrequently.

Pathophysiology of Delayed Ejaculation

Delayed ejaculation usually occurs during sexual intercourse but much less frequently during masturbation. In fact, 85 % of men with either primary or secondary retarded ejaculation are usually able to achieve orgasm through masturbation. This information may be helpful in diagnosing and treating delayed ejaculation. But in some circumstances, delayed ejaculation occurs in both situations; therefore, the man is unable to ejaculate or may only be able to ejaculate after prolonged intercourse or masturbation. This problem can be frustrating and causes distress for both partners involved. In some circumstances, a man can reach pleasurable orgasm without ejaculating semen. This is often referred to as "dry orgasm" (but it must be distinguished from retrograde ejaculation). In a man's experience, orgasm and ejaculation are perceived as identical, but in fact, they are quite separate and distinct processes even though they normally occur about the same time or even simultaneously.

Orgasm is a supremely pleasurable emotional and physical experience, whereas by comparison, ejaculation, even though it is pleasurable, simply represents an unconscious reflex response that is generated by the effective and sexually prolonged stimulation of certain nerves in the genital region.

Orgasm has more associations with the brain than with the pelvis, as is demonstrated, for example, by the fact that orgasm occurs during sleep. Some men have been able to separate and recognize the different parts of the two processes of orgasm and ejaculation, which, on the one side, has let them experience multiple orgasms without having any ejaculation. On the other side, they may have experienced ejaculations with limited feelings of orgasmic pleasure. This information may have bearing on the subject of retarded ejaculation or delayed ejaculation.

Sexual responses are determined and controlled by both the sympathetic and the parasympathetic nervous systems. The sympathetic nervous system generally causes action, and by contrast, the parasympathetic system induces recovery and relaxation. In order for a man's penis to become erect, the smooth muscle fibers of the penile cavities are relaxed so that there can be a flow of blood into the penis. This process is mediated – controlled – by an intricate network of humoral, neurological, and circulatory events; all of which are controlled by the relaxation inducing parasympathetic nervous system. A man's orgasm and his associated ejaculation and the subsequent and consequent relaxation and release of sexual arousal which follows his ejaculation are mostly controlled by the sympathetic nervous system.

The phase of sexual activity known as emission is a parasympathetic nervous system activity, while by contrast, orgasm and ejaculation are actually predominantly under the determination and control of the sympathetic nervous system

Diagnostic Work-Up of Delayed Ejaculation

A detailed medical/psychological/sexual history, as well as a physical (and possibly neurological) examination, the cause of a man's delayed ejaculation, may become clear. In general, somatic and psychosexual causes may be intertwined, but for the sake of diagnostic and therapeutic approach, they must be differentiated.

Somatic Causes

- Medication side effects – Antidepressants, anxiolytic drugs, and antihypertensive medications can slow the ejaculatory response. Retarded ejaculation is estimated to occur in 16–37 % of men taking antidepressant that are selective serotonin reuptake inhibitors. Some research suggests that treatments for erectile dysfunction, such as the PDE-5 inhibitors, sildenafil, vardenafil, and tadalafil, may also cause delayed ejaculation. The other side of the coin is that these medications are used to treat premature ejaculations.
- Hormonal problems such as hypogonadism, hyperthyroidism, hypothyroidism, and an excess of the hormone prolactin.
- Alcohol or illicit drug use.
- Penile problems – chronic inflammation of the penis causing discomfort with intercourse. A nonretractable foreskin often based on sexual ignorance.
- Neurological injuries – Nerve damage caused by strokes and spinal cord injury or conditions such as multiple sclerosis can also create problems with achieving ejaculation. Peripheral neuropathies occur frequently in men with long-standing diabetes mellitus.

Psychological Causes

- Sexual performance anxiety, depression, relationship issues, etc., may cause delayed ejaculation. Psychological factors such as traumatic sexual encounters including sexual abuse, rape, or abuse in the form of incest, and repression of sexual urges and interests due to an excessively repressive sexual environment in the family of origin, often based on religious or cultural beliefs.

- Conditioning by use of unique sexual stimulation may cause men to experience delayed ejaculation while having sexual intercourse with a partner. A man may not gain a sufficient amount of mental or penile stimulation during intercourse to achieve ejaculation. For example, certain sexual fantasies may be lived through while masturbating while these do not come true in actual sexual intercourse. A man may have conditioned himself only in response to a sexual stimulus which cannot be realized in real life. Or a man may be used to masturbating with a very fast motion and may find it difficult to climax with the slower process of intercourse.

It is believed that the majority of delayed ejaculation problems are not somatic in origin since an estimated 85 % of men with either primary or secondary retarded ejaculation are able to achieve orgasm through masturbation. It is likely that these men have no or only a limited somatic problem causing delayed ejaculation but rather a psychological issue needing attention in treatment.

Treatments for Delayed Ejaculation

Obviously, treatment is largely determined by the suspected cause of the problem:

- If a prescribed medication is the suspected cause of a man's retarded ejaculation, find an alternative prescription. Certain essential prescriptions can be replaced in consultation with the prescribing physician.
- Delayed ejaculation and erection problems are very common among excessive drinkers, and they should, without or with professional support, stop or limit drinking. The same applies to users of illicit drugs.
- Inspection of the penis for local lesions or nonretractable foreskin.
- The majority of delayed ejaculation problems seem to be due to psychological causes, and counseling and sex therapy is the primary treatment for restoring complete sexual function. Treatment success varies with the severity of the psychosexual problem. Psychological therapy may gradually resolve a man's sexual anxieties so that he can comfortably climax inside his partner without difficulty. Severe discrepancies between the mental template of a man's sexual arousal and the one of his partner may be more difficult to resolve.

Like with other sexual problems, most men find it awkward to seek professional sexual therapeutic advice, so the ready availability of information and of self-help programs on the internet is helpful. If a man is not able to ejaculate inside the vagina and the couple wishes to have a child, these couples can achieve pregnancy through producing an ejaculate by of electrical stimulation of the prostate area, called electroejaculation, or epididymal extraction of sperms, following which IVF may be carried out to conceive a baby.

Chapter 24
Collection of Bedside Aids for Diagnosis and Tools for Assessment of Treatment to Goal

Peter Huat Chye Lim

Tool for Assessing Premature Ejaculation – The PEDT (Fig. 24.1)

This is a questionnaire to help identity men who may have a problem with ejaculating too soon during sexual activity. Even if you do not have difficulties, please answer all the questions:

- Please mark x the box that best represents you for each of the questions below.
- Please mark only one box for each question.
- Remember there are no right or wrong answers to these questions.
- While your experiences may change from time to time, what we're interested in here is your general experience with intercourse Symonds et al (2002).

Definition

Ejaculation here refers to ejaculation (release of semen) after penetration (when your penis enters your partner).

P.H.C. Lim, MBBS, MMed(Surg), M.Inst.Urol(Lon) FAMS, D.Urol(Lon), FICS
Department of Andrology, Urology Continence Center,
Gleneagles Hospital, Singapore, Singapore

H.T. Naval Medical School, Surabaya, Indonesia

Edith Cowan University, Joondalup, WA, Australia

Society for Men's Health Singapore, Midview City, Singapore

Gleneagles Medical Centre, Singapore, Singapore

Department of Urology, Changi General Hospital, Singapore, Singapore
e-mail: profpeter.lim@gmail.com

P.H.C. Lim (ed.), *Men's Health*,
DOI 10.1007/978-1-4471-4766-4_24,

	Not difficult at all	Somewhat difficult	Moderately difficult	Very difficult	Extremely difficult
1. How difficult is it you to delay ejaculation?	□ 0	□ 1	□ 2	□ 3	□ 4
	Almost never or never 0 %	Less than half the time 25 %	About half the time 50 %	More than half the time 75 %	Almost always or always 100 %
2. Do you ejaculate before you want to?	□ 0	□ 1	□ 2	□ 3	□ 4
3. Do you ejaculate with very little stimulation?	□ 0	□ 1	□ 2	□ 3	□ 4
	Not at all	Slightly	Moderately	Very	Extremely
4. Do you feel frustrated because of ejaculating before you want to?	□ 0	□ 1	□ 2	□ 3	□ 4
5. How concerned are you that your time to ejaculation leaves you partner sexually unfulfilled?	□ 0	□ 1	□ 2	□ 3	□ 4

Fig. 24.1 Premature ejaculation diagnostic tool (PEDT)

Premature Ejaculation Diagnostic Tool (PEDT) Scores

- 5 item, 0–25 score
- Captures the dimension, personal distress and interpersonal distress1
- Sensitivity/specificity analysis suggests that a score ≥11 indicates PE

A PEDT score is obtained by adding the total numbers of these five questions.

- PEDT score ≥11: Has PE
- PEDT score = 9 or 10: Probable PE
- PEDT score ≤ 8: No PE

The use of PEDT has been validated in a study by Symonds.

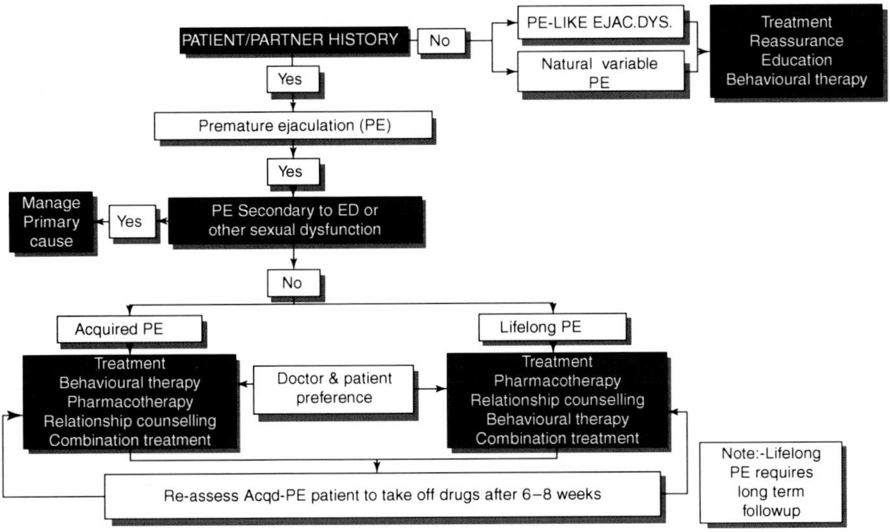

Fig. 24.2 Algorithm for treating PE

Treatment	Advantages	Disadvantages
Behavioural therapy	High reported initial success rate[1]	Limited long-term efficacy[1]
Topical anaesthetics*	Effective in majority of subjects[1]	Penile and vaginal hypoesthesia[2] Female anorgasmia[3] Skin reaction or irritation[3]
Clomipramine*	Significant improvement in IELT[1]	Nausea[1] Erectile dysfunction[4] HSDD[3]
Antidepressant SSRIs*	Significant improvement in IELT[1]	Generally require daily dosing[1,5] Limited data on patient-reported outcomes[1] SSRI withdrawal syndrome[5]
PDE5 inhibitors*	First-line option in PE with concomitant ED[1]	Arguable efficacy only in men with PE[1]
Tramadol*	Significant improvement in IELT[1] Suitable for on-demand dosing[1]	Limited clinical data[1] Limited real-life clinical experience[1] Risk of addiction?[6]

*Off-label use; prescription treatments listed are not approved by Health Authorities for use in PE

1. Gurkan et al.Asian J Androl.2008;10:102-9
2. Morales et al.BJU Int.2007;100:493-501
3. Sharlip.J Sex Med 2005;2(suppL2);103-9
4. Hsu & Shen.Int J Psychiatry Med.1995;25:191-201
5. Hellstrom.Neuropsychiatr Dis Treat.2009;5:37-46
6. Pollice et aL Int J Immunopathol Pharmacol.2008;21: 475-6

Althof et al.(2010) International Society for Sexual Medicine's Guidelines for the Diagnosis and Treatment of Premature Eiaculation.J Sex Med 2010:7:2947-2969

Fig. 24.3 Other off-label drugs used for PE

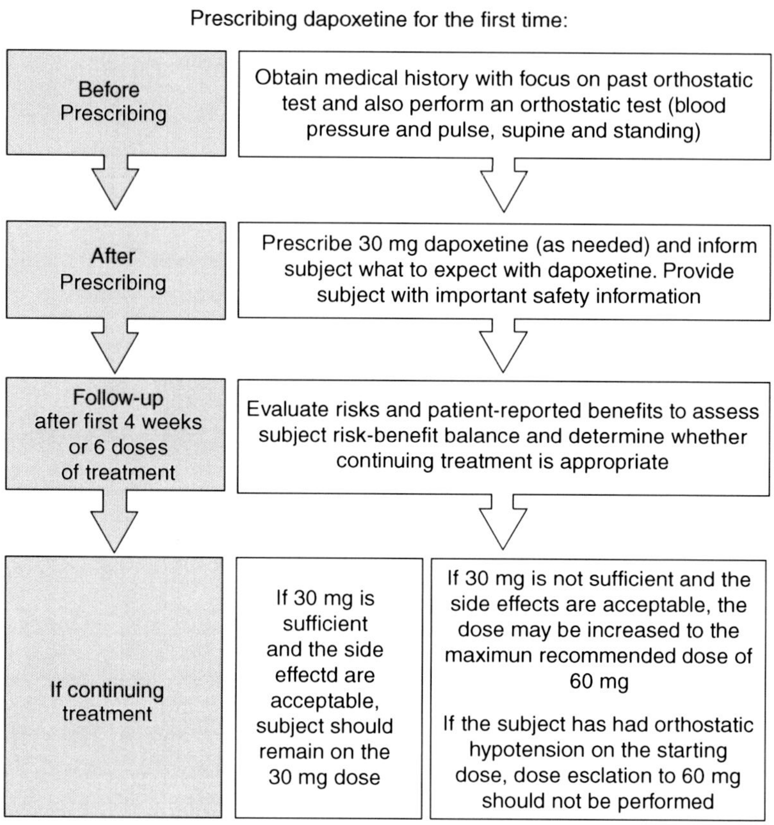

Fig. 24.4 Strategy for first timers using dapoxetine

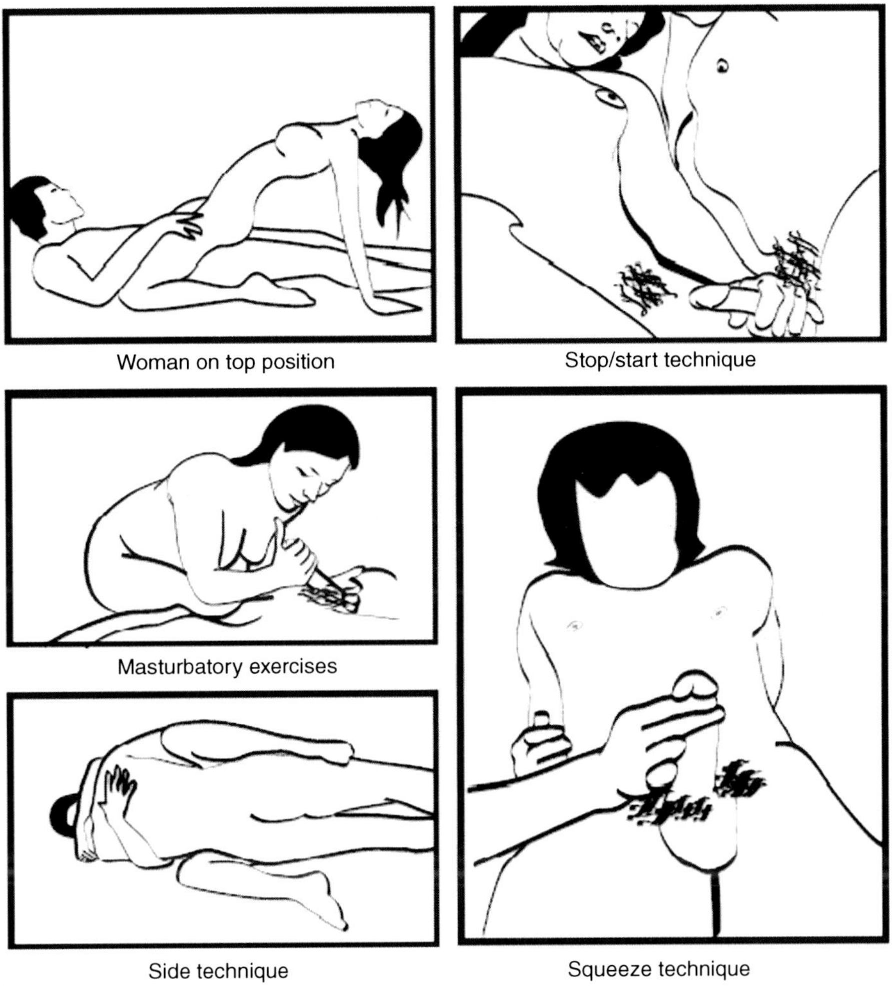

Fig. 24.5 Behavioral techniques for PE

References

Symonds T, Althof SE, Rosen RC, Roblin D, Laytom M. Questionnairre Assessment of Ejaculatory Control; development & validation of a new instrument. Int J Imp Res. 2002;14(4):533. Abstract PS-7-1.

Chapter 25
Frequently Asked Questions on Dapoxetine (FAQ'S)

Peter Huat Chye Lim

Q:
How long does the effect of dapoxetine last?

A:

- Dapoxetine should be taken 1–3 h before sexual activity, no more than once/24 h (Priligy Product Insert).
- Dapoxetine plasma concentrations at 24 h are <5 % of peak levels (Andersson et al. 2006).
- There are no specific pharmacodynamic data about the duration of the effect of dapoxetine.
  - However, clinical data indicates that dapoxetine is effective in men taking dapoxetine up to 3 h before intercourse (Pryor et al. 2006).

P.H.C. Lim, MBBS, MMed(Surg), M.Inst.Urol(Lon) FAMS, D.Urol(Lon), FICS
Department of Andrology, Urology Continence Center,
Gleneagles Hospital, Singapore, Singapore

H.T. Naval Medical School, Surabaya, Indonesia

Edith Cowan University, Joondalup, WA, Australia

Society for Men's Health Singapore, Midview City, Singapore

Gleneagles Medical Centre, Singapore, Singapore

Department of Urology, Changi General Hospital, Singapore, Singapore
e-mail: profpeter.lim@gmail.com

P.H.C. Lim (ed.), *Men's Health*,
DOI 10.1007/978-1-4471-4766-4_25,

Q:
Are there dose restrictions for dapoxetine?

A:

- The recommended starting dose for all men is 30 mg, taken as needed approximately 1–3 h prior to sexual activity.
- The maximum recommended dosing frequency is once every 24 h.
- If the effect of 30 mg is insufficient and the drug is well tolerated, the dose may be increased to the maximum recommended dose of 60 mg.
- If the subject has experienced orthostatic hypotension on the 30 mg dose, dose escalation should not be performed.

Q:
How can you tell that dapoxetine is genuine and not a counterfeit?

A:

- To help physicians verify the authenticity of purchased product:
  - Dapoxetine packs are sealed with a silver tamper-evident sticker.
  - Each pack of dapoxetine has an individual, unique serial number. This can be verified by the subject by visiting a country-specific Janssen website, e.g. www.genuinepriligy.com.sg, and entering the unique 12-digit serial number.
- Serialization and website verification are unique to dapoxetine and are a first for a pharmaceutical product.
- Subjects without internet access can verify the serial number by contacting Janssen.

Q:
How can we avoid or minimize risk of syncope or orthostatic hypotension?

A:

Men should be advised to:

- Take dapoxetine with at least one full glass of water.
- Not to take dapoxetine if they are dehydrated.
- Lie down immediately if they feel faint or light-headed.
- Not to stand up quickly after sitting or lying down for a long time.
- Not to drive or use any tools or machines if they feel faint.
- Inform the doctor if they faint while taking dapoxetine.

Additional Sources of Information

Additional Dapoxetine Sources

Dapoxetine patient leaflets and brochures.

Useful Websites

The European Society for Sexual Medicine. http://www.essm.org/.
The International Society for Sexual Medicine. http://www.issm.info/.
The American Urological Association. http://www.auanet.org/.
The European Men's Health Forum. http://www.emhf.org/.

References

Andersson KE, Mulhall JP, Wyllie MG. Pharmacokinetic and pharmacodynamic features of dapoxetine, a novel drug for "on-demand" treatment of premature ejaculation. BJU Int 2006;97:311–5.

Pryor J, Althof S, Steidle C, Rosen R, Hellstrom W, Shabsigh R, et al. Efficacy and tolerability of dapoxetine in treatment of premature ejaculation: an integrated analysis of two double-blind, randomised controlled trials. Lancet 2006;368:929–37.

Package Leaflet: Information for the user- Priligy Product Insert provided in each box of priligy manufactured. 1–57: Rev 30 Sept 2010 Johnson & Johnson Pte Ltd Singapore.

Part III
Sexually Transmitted Infections

Chapter 26
Overview

Louis Gooren

In the early 1960s, when the "sexual revolution" took off, it seemed that sexually transmitted diseases were of no great concern anymore. There was effective antibiotic treatment which led also to a degree of carelessness among people who engaged in casual sexual encounters. The sequelae of a sexually transmitted disease were no longer the price to pay for the sin of extramarital sex. Over time, herpes genitalis and hepatitis B became problematic because they are in fact incurable. In the early 1980s, AIDS emerged as a hitherto unknown but lethal disease, and over the next years, the mode of transmission was elucidated. Safe sex became mandatory and inescapable. Until then, barrier methods such as condoms had been mainly used for contraceptive purposes. From then on, condoms would be predominantly used for safe sex.

The Human Immunodeficiency Virus (HIV)

- The human immunodeficiency virus is a lentivirus (retrovirus family), and infection, if left untreated, will lead to acquired immunodeficiency syndrome (AIDS), a condition in humans in which the immune system begins to fail, leading to life-threatening opportunistic infections and malignancies. Infection with HIV-1 is associated with a progressive decrease of the $CD4^+$ T cell count. Determination of the patient's $CD4^+$ T cell count and the amount of HIV viral load in the blood are important in disease assessment.

Infection with HIV occurs by transmission of infected blood, semen, vaginal fluid, pre-ejaculate, or breast milk. Within these bodily fluids, HIV is present as

L. Gooren, M.D., Ph.D.
Department of Endocrinology, Free University of Amsterdam, Amsterdam, the Netherlands

H.T. Naval Medical School, Surabaya, Indonesia
e-mail: louisjgooren@gmail.com

P.H.C. Lim (ed.), *Men's Health*,
DOI 10.1007/978-1-4471-4766-4_26, © Springer-Verlag London, 2013

both free virus particles and virus within infected immune cells. The four major routes of transmission are unprotected sexual intercourse, contaminated needles, breast milk, and transmission from an infected mother to her baby during childbirth. Screening of blood products for HIV has largely eliminated transmission through blood transfusions or infected blood products in the developed world.

HIV Infection Has Basically Four Stages

- The four stages of HIV infection are incubation period, acute infection, latency stage, and AIDS. The initial incubation period upon infection is asymptomatic and usually lasts between 2 and 4 weeks. The second stage, acute infection, which lasts an average of 28 days, can include symptoms such as fever, lymphadenopathy (swollen lymph nodes), pharyngitis (sore throat), rash, myalgia (muscle pain), malaise, and mouth and esophageal sores. The latency stage, which occurs third, shows few or no symptoms and can last anywhere from 2 weeks to 20 years and beyond. If left untreated, AIDS, the fourth and final stage of HIV infection develops with onset of various opportunistic infections and malignancies.

There are several strains of the HIV virus, and infection with one strain of HIV does not provide immunity against additional infections with other strains. Superinfection or infection with multiple strains may be associated with more rapid disease progression. Even with early treatment, the risk of HIV transmission still exists. Antiretroviral therapy cannot substitute for prevention measures, such as condom use and safer sex practices.

The majority of HIV infections are acquired through unprotected sexual activity. Sexual transmission can occur when infected sexual secretions of one partner come into contact with the genital, oral, or rectal mucous membranes of another.

HIV has been found at low concentrations in the saliva, tears, and urine of infected individuals, but there are no recorded cases of infection by these secretions, and the potential risk of transmission is negligible.

HIV Treatment

There is currently no vaccine or cure for HIV or AIDS. The only known method of prevention is avoiding exposure to the virus. Current treatment for HIV infection consists of highly active antiretroviral therapy, or HAART. This has been beneficial to many HIV-infected individuals since its introduction in 1996. Current HAART options are combinations (or "cocktails") consisting of at least three drugs belonging to at least two types, or "classes," of antiretroviral agents. In developed countries where HAART is available, doctors assess their patients thoroughly: measuring the viral load, how fast CD4 declines, and patient readiness to commit to lifelong treatment. In general, treatment is considered when CD4 cell counts are less than 500 cells/ul and is recommended when CD4 cell counts are less than 350 cells/ul.

HAART suppresses but does not eradicate the HIV virus. With HAART, many HIV-infected individuals have experienced remarkable improvements in their general health and quality of life, which has led to a large reduction in HIV-associated morbidity and mortality in the developed world. In the absence of HAART, progression from HIV infection to AIDS has been observed to occur at a median of between 9 and 10 years, and the median survival time after developing AIDS is only 9.2 months. In the twenty-first century, with adequate viral suppression and improvements in CD4 cell counts, HIV-infected patients may have a 25–30-year life span. However, HAART sometimes achieves far less than optimal results. This is due to a variety of reasons such as medication intolerance/side effects, prior ineffective antiretroviral therapy, and infection with a drug-resistant strain of HIV. The complexity of these HAART regimens, whether due to pill burden, dosing frequency, meal restrictions, or other issues along with side effects may induce intentional nonadherence. The side effects include lipodystrophy, dyslipidemia, insulin resistance, and increased cardiovascular risks and birth defects. In recent years, the causes of death of HIV-infected individuals are cardiovascular events and malignancy rather than an AIDS-defining diagnosis.

The most effective methods for preventing human immunodeficiency virus (HIV) infection are those that protect against exposure to HIV. Antiretroviral therapy cannot replace behaviors that help avoid HIV exposure. Correct and consistent use of condoms reduces the risk of sexual transmission of HIV by about 85 %.

Safe Sex

Safe sex practices became more urgent in the late 1980s as a result of the AIDS epidemic. Promoting safe sex is now a principal aim of sex education.

Safe sex is the practice of sexual activity in a manner that reduces the risk of infection with sexually transmitted diseases (STDs). Some of these, such as syphilis, gonorrhea, or trichomoniasis can be cured. Others, like AIDS, hepatitis, and herpes simplex are caused by viruses and are hard to cure, or they cannot be cured at all. Condoms can help limit the spread of these diseases. Recently, the use of the term safer sex rather than safe sex has been adopted, on the grounds that risk of transmission of sexually transmitted infections in various sexual activities is a continuum rather than a simple dichotomy between risky and safe.

Much attention has focused on controlling HIV through the use of condoms with intercourse. However, as many STDs can be transmitted through other sexual activities, it is recommended that barrier protection be used for all sexual activities which have the potential for disease transmission, such as manual penetration of the anal or vaginal cavities, or oral stimulation of the genitals.

Safe Sex Precautions

Sex by yourself – Solitary sexual activity is safe. Masturbation, the simple act of stimulating one's own genitalia, is safe so long as contact is not made with other people's discharged bodily fluids.

Modern technology does permit some activities, such as "phone sex" and "cybersex" that allow for partners to engage in sexual activity without being in the same room, eliminating the risks involved with exchanging bodily fluids.

Non-penetrative sex – A range of sex acts, sometimes called "outercourse," can be enjoyed by lovers with significantly reduced risks of infection and pregnancy.

Dangers of Anal Sex

Unprotected anal sex is a high-risk activity regardless of sexual orientation. Research suggests that although gay men are more likely to engage in anal sex, heterosexual couples are more likely not to use condoms when doing so. Anal sex is more risky than vaginal, since the very thin tissues of anus and rectum can be easily damaged during such sex activities as anal intercourse or use of anal toys. Even slight injuries can become "open gates" for various bacteria and viruses, including HIV. This implies that anal sex does require some certain safety measures. First of all, any partner who practices anal sex should be aware of the necessity of using a condom. The condom must be put on properly; otherwise, it does not provide reliable protection. Users should keep in mind that oil-based lubricants damage latex. For this reason, water-based lubricants should be used for anal sex. Those who have allergy to latex should consider use of non-latex condoms, for instance, polyurethane condoms that are compatible with both oil-based and water-based lubricants.

Limiting Fluid Exchange

Various devices are used to avoid contact with blood, vaginal fluid, and semen during sexual activity: condoms cover the penis during sexual activity. They are most frequently made of latex, but can also be made out of polyurethane. Polyurethane is thought to be a safe material for use in condoms, since it is nonporous and viruses cannot pass through it. However, there is less research on its effectiveness than there is on latex.

Condoms

- They are made in different lengths and widths, and different manufacturers produce varying sizes. There is no standard length for condoms, though those made from natural rubber will always stretch, if necessary, to fit the length of the man's

erect penis. The width of a condom can also vary. Some condoms have a slightly smaller width to give a "closer" fit, whereas others will be slightly larger. Condom makers have realized that different lengths and widths are needed and are increasingly broadening their range of sizes. The brand names will be different in each country, so you will need to do your own investigation of different names. There is no particular best brand of condom.
- They may slip off the penis after ejaculation, break due to improper application or physical damage (such as tears caused when opening the package), or break or slip due to latex degradation (typically from usage past the expiration date, improper storage, or exposure to oils). The rate of breakage is between 0.4 and 2.3 %, while the rate of slippage is between 0.6 and 1.3 %. "Double bagging," using two condoms at once, also increases the risk of condom failure.
- Female condoms are inserted into the vagina prior to intercourse. They may also be used for anal sex, although they are less effective.

Medical Gloves – Medical gloves made out of latex, vinyl, nitrile, or polyurethane may be used as a makeshift dental dam during oral sex or to protect the hands during mutual masturbation. Hands may have invisible cuts on them that may admit pathogens that are found in the semen or the vaginal fluids of STD infectees. Although the risk of infection in this manner is thought to be low, gloves can be used as an extra precaution.

Sex Toys – Another way to avoid contact with blood and semen is penetration, but not by the penis, but by such as using (properly cleaned) dildos or other sex toys. If a sex toy is to be used in more than one orifice, a condom can be used over it and changed when the toy is moved. Fisting (penetration by the hand), has its own risks, but the risk of HIV transfer can be reduced by latex gloves or a condom. If a latex barrier is being used, any lubrication must not be oil-based, as this can break down the structure of the latex and undo the protection it gives.

Other Precautions

Acknowledging that it is usually impossible to have entirely risk-free sex with another person, proponents of safe sex recommend that some of the following methods be used to minimize the risks of STD transmission and unwanted pregnancy:

- *Monogamy* or polyfidelity, practiced faithfully, is very safe (as far as STDs are concerned) when all partners are noninfected. However, monogamous people have been infected with sexually transmitted diseases by partners who are sexually unfaithful, have used injection drugs, or were infected by previous sexual partners; the same risks apply to polyfidelitous people, who face slightly higher risks depending on how many people are in the polyfidelitous group.
- *Reducing Number of Partners*: For those who are not monogamous, reducing the number of one's sexual partners, particularly anonymous sexual partners, may also reduce one's potential exposure to STDs. Similarly, one may restrict one's

sexual contact to a community of trusted individuals – this is the approach taken by some nonmonogamous people.

- *Communication* with one's sexual partner(s) makes for greater safety. Before initiating sexual activities, partners may discuss what activities they will and will not engage in and what precautions they will take. This can reduce the chance of risky decisions being made "in the heat of passion."
- *Refraining from the use of recreational drugs*, including alcohol, before and during sexual activity, can protect against associated risks such as lowered inhibitions, decreased immune response, impaired judgment, and loss of consciousness.
- *Regular checkups*: If a person is sexually active with a number of partners, it is important that they get regular sexual health checkups from a doctor. Anyone noticing unusual symptoms should get medical advice quickly as HIV is sometimes asymptomatic or symptoms will have a nonspecific nature and can even be misdiagnosed.
- *Spermicides*: The spermicide nonoxynol-9 has been claimed to reduce the likelihood of STD transmission. However, a recent study by the World Health Organization has shown that nonoxynol-9 is an irritant and can produce tiny tears in mucous membranes, which may increase the risk of transmission by offering pathogens more easy points of entry into the system. Its contraceptive effectiveness is not established and it is not to be promoted.
- *Coitus interruptus* (or "pulling out"), in which the penis is removed from the vagina, anus, or mouth before ejaculation, is not safe sex and can result in STD transmission. Formation of pre-ejaculate, a fluid that oozes from the urethra before actual ejaculation, may contain pathogens such as HIV.
- *Keeping ejaculate fluid out of orifices* will do a great deal to help protect against pregnancy and diseases. Especially important to note if you have cuts in your mouth. In addition, open sores on either partner can permit transmission, as can microscopic breaks in the skin which arise due to friction, or other irregularities in the skin of either partner's genitalia or other body parts.
- *Condoms used with sex toys*. By putting a condom on the sex toy, the user provides better hygiene and prevents transmission of infections if the sex toy is shared. Cleaning of anal sex toys is also a very important matter as many anal sex toys are made of porous materials. Pores retain viruses and bacteria. For this reason, users should clean anal toys (plugs, anal vibrators) thoroughly, preferably with use of special sex toy cleaners. Glass sex toys are more preferred for sexual uses because of their nonporous nature and ability to be sterilized between uses.

Condom Fatigue

"Condom fatigue" or "safe sex fatigue" is a term used to refer to the phenomenon of decreased practice of safe sex, in particular, condom use, over time. Secondly, the "AIDS optimism" hypothesis claims that people have become complacent, following the introduction of more effective drug treatments for AIDS (primarily protease inhibitors), and have lost the sense of danger and urgency surrounding AIDS, and have been reverting to unsafe sex. While antiretroviral treatment has been a major step forward, there is presently no cure for HIV infection and AIDS. Treatment is cumbersome and has substantial side effects which should dim the AIDS optimism to real proportions.

AIDS optimism and condom fatigue might well have generated motives for the new laxness in safe sex practice. Epidemiological rates began to rise about the same time that the protease inhibitors became widespread in the mid to late 1990s.

Condom fatigue can also be used to describe a general weariness of and decreased effectiveness of safer sex messages. In general, the effects of information campaigns on safety and prevention, after their initial shock effect, wear off in the course of time ("prevention fatigue").

Conclusion

A fact of life is that STI still strikes and often it does so. Thus, there is still a place for a pocket compendium for the busy nonspecialist which can be used as a quick aide-memoire for diagnosis and treatment regimens currently being used for the common sexually transmitted diseases. The usual texts are so detailed that no ordinary practitioner would have the time to reference these during a busy morning ward round in the hospital or at the average 5–10 min consultations at the general practitioner's office. As the Chief Editor of this book called it, this text fulfills its intended objective of being truly an Idiot's Guidebook for the ordinary practitioner or a Hitchhikers Guide and Companion when confronted with sexually transmitted diseases which he does see often and must manage in his everyday practice

Bibliography

Adler M, Cowan F, French P, editors. ABC of sexually transmitted infections. 5th ed. BMJ Publ. Group, London, 2004. ISBN 0-7279-17517.

Daniel T. Presentation of disturbing trends in Singapore of young people attending an STI Clinic. Singapore SexPo conference, 2006.

Special Focus Profiles, trends, distribution of STDs and HIV & prevention programs with consequences in women, infants, adolescents, young, adults, minorities, MSM, & persons entering correction facilities: Div of STD Prevention NCHSTP, CDC, Sexually transmitted disease surveillance 2006/2007. 23–166.

Lim KB, et al. Chlamydial infection in female prostitutes in Singapore. Med J. 1989; 30(3):263–4.

Chapter 27
HIV/AIDS

Peter Huat Chye Lim and Sin Yew Wong

Introduction

HIV-AIDS is an infection caused by the human immunodeficiency virus (HIV). Virus and host factors determine development of symptomatic HIV infection and AIDS.

Transmission: Sexual contact (virus present in the semen or the vaginal fluid), blood borne (contaminated syringes, transfusion of blood products), and mother-to-child transmission.

Signs and Symptoms: Acute infection lasts 1–8 weeks characterized by viremia, fever, sore throat, and enlarged lymph nodes. During the acute stage, there is often intense viremia, and the patient is highly infectious. Asymptomatic stage begins several months after acute infection and lasts 1–10 years depending on the immune response. There is steady depletion of the immune system with gradual decrease in CD 4 cell counts often coupled with increasing HIV viral load. It is essentially a multisystem disease related to a depleted immune system: fatigue, diarrhea, weight loss, generalized persistent lymphadenopathy, anorexia, and night sweats may develop and opportunistic infections occur, heralding the onset of AIDS.

P.H.C. Lim, MBBS, MMed(Surg), M.Inst.Urol(Lon) FAMS, D.Urol(Lon), FICS
Department of Andrology, Urology Continence Center,
Gleneagles Hospital, Singapore, Singapore

H.T. Naval Medical School, Surabaya, Indonesia

Edith Cowan University, Joondalup, WA, Australia

Society for Men's Health Singapore, Midview City, Singapore

Gleneagles Medical Centre, Singapore, Singapore

Department of Urology, Changi General Hospital, Singapore, Singapore
e-mail: profpeter.lim@gmail.com

S.Y. Wong, MBBS, MMed(Int Med), FAMS (✉)
Gleneagles Medical Centre, Gleneagles Hospital, Singapore, Singapore

P.H.C. Lim (ed.), *Men's Health*,
DOI 10.1007/978-1-4471-4766-4_27, © Springer-Verlag London, 2013

Common AIDS-Defining Illnesses

- Cryptococcal meningitis
- PTB or extrapulmonary TB
- Kaposi's sarcoma
- Cerebral toxoplasmosis
- Candidiasis of the esophagus
- Salmonella bacteremia
- Cerebral lymphoma
- CMV retinitis

Differences in Developed/Developing Countries (AIDS-Defining Diseases)

Developed World:

Pneumococcal pneumonia
Esophageal candidiasis
Non-Hodgkin's lymphoma
TB (lung and extrapulmonary)
TB (lung and extrapulmonary)
HIV wasting syndrome
Cerebral toxoplasmosis
Cryptococcal meningitis

Lab Diagnosis

Test for HIV should be offered to all persons with behavioral risk factors, tuberculosis, invasive pneumococcal disease, etc. Infected individuals develop HIV antibodies within 1–4 months after infection that can be detected by:

- Enzyme immunoassay serum antibodies, e.g., ELISA screening test
- Confirmation with western blot technique if screening ELISA is reactive

Diagnosis of acute HIV infection is confirmed by a positive virus detection assay (plasma HIV RNA, cellular proviral DNA) in the presence of a negative or evolving (rising) antibody profile.

Treatment

- Counseling and psychological support as there is often social stigma and discrimination
- Prophylaxis and treatment of opportunistic infections

- The initiation of antiretroviral therapy is largely dependent on the CD4 cell count with values less than 500 cells/ul as starting points for consideration

Antiretroviral therapy guidelines are updated regularly by the International AIDS Society and other medical societies/national institutions. Treatment should only be initiated by physicians who are experienced and familiar with the management of this complex disease.

Prevention and Control

- Surveillance
- Counseling and health education
- Safe blood supply
- Strategies to reduce high-risk behavior in targeted populations
- Antiretroviral therapies to reduce mother-to-child transmission
- Protection of healthcare staff
- Treatment and control of other STIs

Recommendation for HIV Antibody Testing

In those practicing high-risk sexual behavior, i.e.:

- Having casual partners
- Having multiple partners
- Having sex with a partner whose STI/HIV status you are unsure of
- Having sex with a spouse/steady partner who may not be faithful to you or have been practicing high-risk sexual practices

Value of HIV Testing

1. Protection of current or future sexual partners and the prevention of vertical transmission
2. Access to preventive and therapeutic care including antiretroviral drugs where applicable
3. Allows life decisions to be made
4. Resolves anxiety, especially in those at low risk

Disadvantages

1. Psychological impact of dealing with the diagnosis
2. Discrimination, social stigma, and impact on relationships
3. Employment and financial implications

Miscellaneous Needlestick Injuries in Staff

Combination antiretroviral therapy should start as soon as possible after the exposure incident – best within 24 h for duration of 4 weeks.

Bibliography

Adler M, Cowan F, French P, Mitchell H, Richens J. ABC of sexually transmitted infections. 5th ed. BMJ Publishing; 2004.

Clutterbuck D. Specialist training in sexually transmitted infections & HIV. Edinburgh/London/New York: Elsevier/Mosby; 2004.

European Study Group on Heterosexual Transmission of HIV. Comparison of female to male and male to female transmission of HIV in 563 stable couples. BMJ. 1992;304(6830):809–13. PMID 1392708.

HIV in the United Kingdom 2012. http://www.hpa.org.uk/webw/HPAweb&Page&HPAwebAutoListName/Page/1200660065903?p=1200660065903.

Leynaert B, Downs AM, de Vincenzi I. Heterosexual transmission of human immunodeficiency virus: variability of infectivity throughout the course of infection. European Study Group on Heterosexual Transmission of HIV. Am J Epidemiol. 1998;148(1):88–96. PMID 9663408.

Pattan R, Snow M, Handy P, Sankar KN, Elawad B, editors. Oxford handbook of genitourinary medicine, HIV & aids. Oxford University Press; 2005.

Peate I. Manual of sexually transmitted infections. London/Philadelphia: Whurr Publ; 2005.

Varghese B, Maher JE, Peterman TA, Branson BM, Steketee RW. Reducing the risk of sexual HIV transmission: quantifying the per-act risk for HIV on the basis of choice of partner, sex act, and condom use. Sex Transm Dis. 2002;29(1):38–43. PMID 11773877.

Chapter 28
Breaking the News and Counseling

Elias Tak Chuen Tam

The counseling tasks of the family doctor in testing STDs include:

1. Breaking the "bad news" sensitively to the patients
2. Supporting the patient and the family emotionally by dispelling myths and referring them to the relevant centers for further counseling, test, or treatment when necessary

Pre-counseling Preparation

To be effective in achieving the above tasks, the family doctor needs to prepare the following:

1. *Brochures on STDs* in various languages are available from DSC. For brochures, write to "Information officer I/C, DSC clinic, block 31, Kelantan Lane, Singapore 200031."
2. Contact for nearby family service counseling center.
3. *Infectious Diseases Act* (Chapter 137) (#).

First Encounter

During the same consultation when the test is being taken, it is important to find out and write down the following points on R.I.C.E:

R – reason for encounter (why is he/she taking the test? Any recent exposure? Symptoms?)
I – idea (what does he/she understand STDs to be?)

E.T.C. Tam, MBBS, GDFM, GD(FP) Dermatology
EHA Clinic, Shaw Centre, Singapore

P.H.C. Lim (ed.), *Men's Health*,
DOI 10.1007/978-1-4471-4766-4_28, © Springer-Verlag London 2013

C – concern (what is the main worry?)
E – expectation (what does he/she hope to achieve?)

Breaking the Bad News

1. Be nonjudgmental and sympathetic. Maintain eye contact.
2. Inform the results, and explain the significance of it. The brochure that you have prepared will be most helpful.
3. Give the patient a moment to let the message sink in.
4. Explain the treatments available. For viral infection that cannot be cured, explain the strategies to control it, such as prophylactic Acyclovir for frequent attacks of herpes simplex.

Counseling

1. If other possible STDs have not been tested, it is important to explain the need to screen for them.
2. Explain the importance of abstinence till cure is confirmed to prevent the STD from spreading (or using condoms if not possible to abstain).
3. Explain the need to test and treat his partner(s) to prevent further spread and reinfection.
4. You may need to break your counseling into more than one session. The patient may not be ready to take in too much information especially after just receiving the "bad" news.
5. When appropriate, take the opportunity to share with the patient strategies to reduce risk of reinfection. This includes proper use of condoms, including oral and anal sex, and avoidance of multiple sexual partners or persons with multiple partners.
6. Check with patients on their beliefs of safe sex. Correct misconceptions such as "use of coke as a wash after sex can prevent STD," "young girl will not have STD," or "taking antibiotic from 'street vendor' after sex to protect from STD."
7. For those with high-risk behavior but tested negative, it is prudent to explain the need for retest at 1 month, 3 months, and 6 months after last exposure in case of initial false negative result.
8. For those undergoing treatment, emphasize the importance of "test of cure" after treatment as resistance to treatment is not uncommon.
9. For cases that need to be referred to a specialist or DSC, such as HIV infection, extra time is needed to reassure the patient that appropriate treatment will improve the outcome significantly.

The issue of contact tracing is very sensitive as the fear of marital breakdown is very real.

Infectious diseases act (Chapter 137)

Part IV
Control of aids and HIV infection
Protection of identity of person with AIDS, HIV Infection or other sexually transmitted disease

25 (1) Any person who, in the performance or exercise of his functions or duties under this Act, is aware or has reasonable grounds for believing that another person has AIDS or HIV Infection or is suffering from a sexually transmitted disease or is a carrier of that disease shall not disclose any information which may identify the other person except -

(a) with the consent of the other person;
(b) when it is necessary to do so in connection with the administration or execution of anything under this Act;
(c) when ordered to do so by a court;
(d) to any medical practitioner or other health staff who is treating or caring for the other person;
(e) to any blood, organ, semen or breast milk bank that has received or will receive any blood, organ, semen or breast milk from the other person;
(f) for statistical reports and epidemiological purposes if the information is used in such a way that the identity of the other person is not made known;
(g) to the victim of a sexual assault by the other person;
(h) to the Controller of Immigration for the purposes of the Immigration Act (Cap. 133);
(i) to the next-of-kin of the other person upon the death of such person;
(j) to any person or class of persons to whom, in the opinion of the Director, it is in the public interest that the information be given; or
(k) when authorised by the Minister to publish such information for the purposes of public health or public safety. *[5/92;13/99]*

(2) Any person who contravenes subsection (1) shall be guilty of an offence and shall be liable on conviction to a fine not exceeding $2,000 or to imprisonment for a term not exceeding 3 months or to both. *[5/92]*

(3) For the purposes of subsection (1) (a), the consent of the other person includes -

Fig. 28.1 Relevant section from the infectious diseases act from Ministry of health Singapore

The patient may request that the spouse or partner not to be told of the real reason for coming down to see you. Often, the partner may suspect the real reason but choose to play dumb. Sometimes, the couple may break down and cry.

There may be much deeper issues within the family, and a referral to the nearest family service counseling center may be useful for the couple.

With regard to the issue of confidentiality, all doctors must get to know the Infectious Diseases Act, Chapter 137 (see Figs. 28.1 and 28.2)

It is best to convince the patient to agree to provide his contact and the possible need to reveal his condition to his/her partner(s). In the case of serious infection such as HIV, if the risk to his partner is too high, you may want to contact the director of medical services of MOH to get approval to inform the spouse despite his refusal of consent.

MD 131

INFECTIOUS DISEASES ACT
(CHAPTER 137)

Regulation 2

INFECTIOUS DISEASES (NOTIFICATION OF INFECTIOUS DISEASES) REGULATIONS

NOTIFICATION OF INFECTIOUS DISEASES UNDER SECTION 6

PARTICULARS OF PATIENT (Please ✓ appropriate box where applicable)

Name of Patient (BLOCK LETTERS) | NRIC No./Passport No./Foreign Identification Number (FIN)

Gender: ☐ Male ☐ Female | Date of Birth (dd/mm/yyyy) | Ethnic Group: ☐ Chinese ☐ Indian ☐ Malay ☐ Others | Residential Status: ☐ Resident ☐ Non-Resident | Occupation

Residential Address | Postal Code | Telephone No. Home

Place of Work/School/Child Care Centre/Kindergarten | Office/HP/PG

DISEASE DIAGNOSED (CLINICAL OR LABORATORY DIAGNOSIS)

TO CD@ **NOT LATER THAN 24 HOURS** FROM TIME OF DIAGNOSIS. FAX NO. 62215528 OR 62215538

☐ 1. Avian influenza
☐ 2. Cholera
☐ 3. Dengue
☐ 4. Dengue haemorrhagic fever
☐ 5. Encephalitis
☐ 6. Hand, foot and mouth disease
☐ 7. Legionellosis
☐ 8. Malaria
☐ 9. Nipah virus infection
☐ 10. Paratyphoid
☐ 11. Plague
☐ 12. SARS
☐ 13. Typhoid
☐ 14. Yellow fever
☐ ✧ 15. Others (Specify) ____________

✧ For any disease not appearing in this form,which may be of an infectious nature and result in an epidemic. If name of disease is not known, please specify symptoms.

TO CD@ **NOT LATER THAN 72 HOURS** FROM TIME OF DIAGNOSIS FAX NO. 62215528 OR 62215538

☐ #16. Chickenpox
☐ #17. Diphtheria
☐ 18. Hepatitis, viral
☐ #19. Measles
☐ #20. Mumps
☐ #21. Poliomyelitis
☐ #22. Rubella

 # For notifiable diseases marked #, please provide vaccination history :

☐ Yes - If yes, Date of vaccination (dd/mm/yyyy)
☐ No

TO DCE¶ **NOT LATER THAN 72 HOURS** FROM TIME OF DIAGNOSIS. FAX NO. 62541616

☐ 23. AIDS
☐ 24. HIV infection (non-AIDS)
☐ **25. Tuberculosis

***** For tuberculosis, the Tuberculosis Notification Form MD 532-92 should also be completed.***

TO DSC✖ **NOT LATER THAN 72 HOURS** FROM TIME OF DIAGNOSIS. FAX NO. 62994335

☐ *26. Chancroid
☐ *27. Gonorrhoea
☐ *28. Non-gonococcal urethritis
☐ *29. Non-infectious syphilis (latent/tertiary)✧
☐ *30. Infectious syphilis (primary/secondary)✧
☐ *31. Congenital syphilis
☐ *32. Genital herpes (first episode)
☐ *33. Genital herpes (recurrent)
☐ 34. Leprosy

** For sexually transmitted infections marked *, full name, NRIC/Passport No./FIN, address and telephone number need not be completed. Initials of the patient should be given.*

✧ Circle as appropriate

Diagnosis: ☐ Clinical ☐ Confirmed by laboratory tests

Date present diagnosis was made/ suspected (dd/mm/yyyy)

Date of onset of illness (dd/mm/yyyy)

Follow-up of patient
☐ Treated as outpatient
☐ Referred to Communicable Disease Centre
☐ Referred to Dept of STI Control Clinic, Kelantan Lane
☐ Others (specify) ....

Travel history over the past one month
From (dd/mm/yyyy) to Countries visited : ....

PARTICULARS OF INFORMANT

Name of Medical Practitioner/Scientist (BLOCK LETTERS) | Signature and Date | Physician Code (MCR No.)

Name and Address of Clinic/Hospital/Institution/Laboratory | Telephone Number

EXPLANATORY NOTES

@ CD : Deputy Director of Medical Services (E&DC), Communicable Diseases Division, Ministry of Health, 16 College Road, Singapore 169854, Tel: 1800-3258451 (Toll free line), 63258357, 63258358, Fax : 62215528 / 62215538

¶ DCE : Head, Department of Clinical Epidemiology, Communicable Disease Centre, Tan Tock Seng Hospital, 142 Moulmein Road, Singapore 308087, Tel: 62568123, Fax : 62541616

✖ DSC : Head, Department of STI Control Clinic, Blk 31 Kelantan Lane #02-16, Singapore 200031, Tel: 62939648, Fax : 62994335

1. Notification is required in accordance with section 6 of the Infectious Diseases Act.
2. This notification form should be used whenever a notifiable infectious disease is diagnosed or suspected in a clinic, hospital or laboratory.

12.12.2005

Fig. 28.2 Mandatory STI notification form for medical practitioners in Singapore

Where to find the nearby or appropriate counseling center:

1. DSC
   (a) Able to assist in providing brochures, contact tracing, anonymous HIV testing and counseling
   (b) Tel. 62399648
   (c) Pre-recorded information – 62952944
   (d) AIDS/STI hotline – 1800–2521324 or 62946300
   (e) www.dsc-sexualhealth.com.sg/
   (f) 31 Kelantan Lane #01-16, Singapore 200031
2. MCYS (Ministry of Community Development, Youth and Sports)
   (a) Website provides search engine for the family center by region, name, or address of center and services available
   (b) www.mcys.gov.sg
3. Centre for Fathering Limited
   (a) Provide family counseling as well as activities to help father bond with family
   (b) Tel. 62558408
   (c) www.fatheringmatters.com

Recommended opportunistic STD screening includes:

1. HIV
2. Syphilis
3. Hepatitis B

Avoid routine screening tests that are not of significant value, e.g., serology test for chlamydia and gonorrhea (perform culture from appropriate site if indicated) and serology test for herpes simplex (HSV) in asymptomatic patients, especially the old serology test that cannot reliably distinguish HSV-1 and HSV-2.

Bibliography

How to tell your girlfriend you have an STD. Accessed on 6 Dec 2012.

E-Cards let you break the news anonymously. Accessed on 6 Dec 2012.

Chapter 29
Prostatitis in Men

Ho Siew Hong and Peter Huat Chye Lim

Introduction

- Common but confusing
- Affects adult males
- Patients are unhappy with treatment, clinicians are frustrated
- Occurs in several distinct forms and syndromes
- Recognition of these patterns would result in better treatment results

Classification of Prostatitis

Traditional, Drach 1978

- Acute bacterial
- Chronic bacterial
- Chronic nonbacterial
- Prostatodynia

H.S. Hong, MBBS, MMed(Surg), FRCS, FAMS (✉)
Ho Urological Clinic, Gleneagles Medical Centre, Gleneagles Hospital, Singapore, Singapore
e-mail: siewhongho@yahoo.com.sg

P.H.C. Lim, MBBS, MMed(Surg), M.Inst.Urol(Lon) FAMS, D.Urol(Lon), FICS
Department of Andrology, Urology Continence Center,
Gleneagles Hospital, Singapore, Singapore

H.T. Naval Medical School, Surabaya, Indonesia

Edith Cowan University, Joondalup, WA, Australia

Society for Men's Health Singapore, Midview City, Singapore

Gleneagles Medical Centre, Singapore, Singapore

Department of Urology, Changi General Hospital, Singapore, Singapore

P.H.C. Lim (ed.), *Men's Health*,
DOI 10.1007/978-1-4471-4766-4_29, © Springer-Verlag London 2013

National Institutes of Health, Krieger 1999

- Acute bacterial
- Chronic bacterial
- Chronic prostatitis/chronic pelvic pain syndrome
  - (a) Inflammatory
  - (b) Noninflammatory
- Asymptomatic inflammatory prostatitis

Acute Bacterial Prostatitis

- Acute onset
- Tender and swollen prostate on DRE
- Signs of general illness – fever and chills
- Urinary tract infection
- Inflammatory cells in prostatic secretions
- Positive culture – blood, urine, or prostatic secretions

Chronic Bacterial Prostatitis

- Subtle
- Relapsing recurrent UTIs
- No signs of systemic infection
- Mildly or non-tender prostate on DRE
- Inflammatory cells in prostatic secretions
- Persistence of bacteria in prostatic secretions, i.e., positive culture

Chronic Prostatitis: Inflammatory

- Chronic nonbacterial prostatitis
- Pain
- No history of UTI
- Minimal signs on DRE
- >10 hpf leukocytes in prostatic secretions
- Negative culture on urine and prostatic secretions

Chronic Prostatitis: Noninflammatory

- Prostatodynia
- Persistent pain
- No history of UTI and absence of physical signs
- Absence of inflammation cells or bacteria in urine or prostatic secretions

Asymptomatic Inflammatory Prostatitis

- Histological proof of chronic prostatitis without clinical symptoms of pain or disease

Etiology and Pathogenesis

Four main etiologies for induction:

- Bacteria
- Urine reflux
- Immunological status of host and adherence capacity of infective agents
- Psychic aspect
  Chronicity of the process depends on balances between predisposing factors and/or host defense.

Bacterial Component

- Undisputed in type I and II
- Common strains – *E. coli*, Proteus, Klebsiella, Enterobacter, Pseudomonas
- Questionable in type III and IV
- Possibly Cryptic infections – trichomonas, fungi, chlamydia, mycoplasma, viruses

Urine Reflux

- Intraprostatic urinary reflux occurs commonly; probably plays an important role in the pathogenesis of bacterial prostatitis (type I and II)
- Intraprostatic urinary reflux may cause "chemical" prostatitis in type III and IV

Host Versus Pathogen

- Chronic prostatitis as a result of altered immunity due to an antigenic stimulus*
- Immunological status of host and the adherence capacity of the infective pathogen play a role in the result of treatment and development of a chronic state

Psychic Aspect

- Importance of mental stress has been underestimated*
- NIH classification recognizes pain as the leading symptom, together with a wide range of voiding, psychological, and sexual disturbances

Method of Diagnosis

- Evaluation is a complicated task as there is lack of a clearly objective and measurable parameter
- "Inflammation of the prostate"
- Inflammation is an accompaniment to an infection, but not all inflammatory reactions can be explained by an infection

Symptoms

- Pain – lower abdomen, perineal, scrotal, inguinal, and penile
- Voiding disturbances
- Temporary sexual dysfunction
- Mental distress

History

- Urinary tract infection
- Sexually transmitted disease
- Urological procedures
- Host defense (DM, immunosuppression)

Physical Examination

- Abdominal, inguinal, scrotum, penile, and perineal areas
- Digital rectal examination (DRE)

Investigations

- Urine analysis and culture
- Cystoscopy and upper urinary tract imaging in the presence of hematuria
- Stamey "four-glass test" – well known but seldom used
- Nickel's pre-massage and post-massage test
- Semen studies
- PSA
- TRUS ± biopsy
- Uroflow studies

Stamey "Four-Glass Test"

- "Golden standard"
- To differentiate types of prostatitis
- VB1 1st void urine – urethra
- VB2 midstream urine – bladder
- EPS – prostate
- VB3 post-massage urine – prostate

Nickel's Pre-massage and Post-massage Test

- Pre-M: midstream urine
- Post-M: after DRE
- Comparison between post-M and pre-M
- Leukocytosis >10 hpf or a one log higher
- Significant bacteruria> 10 or a one log higher

Semen Studies

- Leukocyte count> 10 hpf
- Cultures

Prostate Specific Antigen (PSA)

- Can be elevated in prostatitis
- PSA "leak" in prostatitis
- Not specific or diagnostic
- Release of other inflammatory agents, e.g., cytokines and TNF

TRUS ± Biopsy

- No specific findings on TRUS
- Suggestions: irregular internal echoes, edema, increased blood flow, calcifications, and ejaculatory duct obstruction
- Targeted biopsy (cyst, abscess)
- Random biopsy not encouraged

Uroflow and Urodynamic Studies

- Obstructed voiding

Treatment

Acute Bacterial Prostatitis

- Antibiotics – trimethoprim-sulfamethoxazole, fluoroquinolone, aminoglycoside, cephalosporin
- Hydration
- Analgesia
- Antipyretics
- Stool softener
- Suprapubic catheter drainage in ARU

Chronic Bacterial Prostatitis

- Bactrim, fluoroquinolones
- Duration: 3–16 weeks

- Infections that are not cured – continuous, suppressive, low-dose antibiotics, e.g., Bactrim 1/1 om and nitrofurantoin 100 mg om
- TURP in patients that cannot be cured by medical therapy, esp. with infected prostatic stones

Chronic Prostatitis/Chronic Pelvic Pain Syndrome

- Plenty of men with the condition
- Defined mainly by symptoms
- Clinical problem: chronic long-standing symptoms not improved with antimicrobial therapy
- Median age: 43 years
- Significant not necessarily related to urination
- Pain in perineum; often worse after ejaculation
- Significant urinary symptoms

Principles of Therapy

Always start with 1st line antibiotics, alpha-blockers, and anti-inflammatory drugs. Symptoms needing additional attention include pain and voiding symptoms. If this treatment does not work, proceed to the other add-ons:

Complete therapeutic repertoire at clinician's disposable:

- Alpha-blockers – improve voiding dysfunction, decreases intraprostatic reflux
- Incremental dose and maintain for at least 6 months, if not indefinitely
- Counseling and patient education
- Hot sitz bath – symptomatic relief
- For "pain" a short course with NSAIDS useful. May need amitriptyline, Neurontin, tizanidine, or opiates
- Anticholinergic drugs if patient has voiding dysfunction
- Possibly antibiotics
- Prostatic massage only useful when the prostate is "congested"
- Tension myalgia of pelvic floor – diazepam
- Stress management by psychologist or psychiatrist
- No dietary restriction unless an irritative substance is identified, e.g., spicy food and alcohol

Newer therapeutic strategies include:

- Combined antibiotic alpha-blocker therapy
- Embrel – antibody to TNF alpha
- Elmiron Sulfate

- Proscar/Avodart
- Thermotherapy/TUNA (transurethral Needle ablation of prostate) 50–70 % better
- Botox type A injections into the prostate – this is currently the favorite
- Electromagnetic stimulation of the pelvic floor

Summary

- Complex set of conditions
- Not fully understood
- Important to classify accurately
- Treatment according to subtype
- Multi-aspect approach, esp. chronic prostatitis/chronic pelvic pain syndrome

Bibliography

Collins MM, Stafford RS, O'Leary MP, et al. How common is prostatitis? A national survey of physician visits. J Urol. 1998;159:1224–8.

Drach DW. Sexuality and prostatitis: a hypothesis. J Am Vener Dis Assoc. 1976;3:87–9.

Litwin M, McNaughton-Collins M, Fowler FJ, and the Chronic Prostatitis Collaborative Research Network, et al. The National Institutes of Health Chronic Prostatitis Symptom Index: development and validation of a new outcome measure. J Urol. 1999;162:369–75.

Meares EM. Prostatitis and related disorders. In: Walsh P et al., editors. Campbell's urology. 7th ed. Philadelphia: WB Saunders; 1998. p. 615–29.

Mehik A, Hellstrom P, Lukkarinen O, et al. Epidemiology of prostatitis in Finnish men: a population-based cross-sectional study. BJU Int. 2000;86:443–8.

Moon TD, Hagen L, Heisey DM. Urinary symptomatology in younger men. Urology. 1997;50:700–3.

National Institutes of Health Summary Statement. National Institute of Health/National Institute of Diabetes and Digestive and Kidney Diseases workshop on chronic prostatitis. Executive Summary, Bethesda, 1995.

Nickel JC. Prostatitis and related conditions. In: Walsh PC, Wein AJ, Vaughan Jr ED, Retik AB, editors. Campbell's urology. 8th ed. Philadelphia: WB Saunders Company; 2002.

Nickel JC, Downey J, Hunter D, Clark J. Prevalence of prostatitis like symptoms in a population based study employing the NIH Chronic Prostatitis Symptom Index (NIH-CPSI). J Urol. 2001;165:842–5.

Roberts RO, Lieber MM, Bostwick DG, et al. A review of clinical and pathological prostatitis syndromes. Urology. 1997;49:809–21.

Evaluation

Collins MM, Stafford RS, O'Leary MP, Barry MJ. How common is prostatitis? A national survey of physician visits. J Urol. 1998;159:1224–8.

Collins MM, O'Leary MP, Litwin MS, Calhoun EA, et al. Quality of life is impaired in men with chronic prostatitis: results from the NIH cohort study. J Urol. 2000;163(suppl):23 (abstract).

Gushchin B, Francis ME. Epidemiological data on the prevalent diagnostic and treatment procedures for chronic prostatitis in the ambulatory care setting. In: Abstract paper presented at the 3rd international prostatitis collaborative network, Washington, D.C., 23–25 Oct 2000, p. 29.
Krieger JN, Egan KJ, Ross SO, Jacobs R, Berger RE. Chronic pelvic pains represent the most prominent urogenital symptoms of "chronic prostatitis". Urology. 1996;48:715–21.
Nadler RB, Koch AE, Calhoun E, et al. IL-1B and TNF-α in prostatic secretions are indicators in the evaluation of men with chronic prostatitis. J Urol. 2000;164:214–8.
Nickel JC. Prostatitis: evolving management strategies. Urol Clin North Am. 1999;26:737–51.
Shoskes DA, Mazurick C, Landis R, Ruggieri MR, et al. Bacterial cultures in urine, prostatic fluid and semen of men with chronic pelvic pain syndrome: role of culture for 2 vs 5 days. J Urol. 2000;163(suppl):24 (abstract).

Treatment

Antibiotics

Bjerkland-Johansen T, Gruneberg RN, Guibert J, et al. The role of antibiotics in the treatment of chronic prostatitis: a consensus statement. Eur Urol. 1998;34:457–66.
Giannopoulos A, Korzantis G, et al. Pharmacokinetics of Clarithromycin in the prostate: implications for the treatment of chronic abacterial prostatitis. J Urol. 2001;165:97–9.
Naber KG, Busch W, Focht J. Ciprofloxacin in the treatment of chronic bacterial prostatitis: a prospective, non-comparative multicenter clinical trial with long term followup. Int J Antimicrob Agents. 2000;14:143–9.
Simmons PD, Thin RN. Minocycline in chronic abacterial prostatitis: a double blind prospective trial. Br J Urol. 1985;57:43–5.
Weidner W, Ludwig M, Brahler E, Schiefer HG. Outcome of antibiotic therapy with ciprofloxacin in chronic bacterial prostatitis. Drugs. 1999;58 suppl 2:103–6.

Alpha-Blockers

Barbalias GA, Nikiforidis G, Liatsikos EN. Alpha-blockers for the treatment of chronic prostatitis in combination with antibiotics. J Urol. 1998;159(3):883–7.
Neal DE, Moon TD. Use of terazosin in prostatodynia and validation of a symptom score questionnaire. Urology. 1994;43:460–5.
Osborn DE, George NJ, Rao PN, Barnard RJ, Reading C, Marklow C, et al. Prostatodynia-physiological characteristics and rational management with muscle relaxants. Br J Urol. 1981;53:621–3.

Anti-inflammatory Medication

Canale D, Turchi P, Giorgi PM, Scaricabarozzi I, Menchini-Fabris GF. Treatment of abacterial prostato-vesiculitis with nimesulide. Drugs. 1993;4 suppl 1:147–50.
Muraro G. Clinical study on the efficacy and safety of seaprose S combined with local prostate hyperthermia in chronic nonbacterial prostatitis. Controlled study versus local prostatic hyperthermia. Arch Med Interna. 1995;47:73–86.

Nickel JC, Gittleman M, Malek G, Moon T, Murdock M, Tomera K, Pontari M, et al. Rofecoxib in the treatment of chronic nonbacterial prostatitis: a phase II randomized placebo controlled study. In: Abstract paper presented at the 3rd international prostatitis collaborative network, Washington, D.C., 23–25 Oct 2000, p. 25.

Other Therapies

Clemens JQ, Nadler RB, Schaeffer AJ, Bushman W. Biofeedback, pelvic floor reeducation and bladder training for chronic pelvic pain syndrome in males. J Urol. 2000;163(suppl): 26 (abstract).

Kaplan SA, Te AE, Jacobs BZ. Urodynamic evidence of vesical neck obstruction in men with misdiagnosed chronic nonbacterial prostatitis and the therapeutic role of endoscopic incision of the bladder neck. J Urol. 1994;152:2063–5.

Kaplan SA, Santarosa RP, D'Alisera PM, Fay BJ, Ikeguchi EF, Hendricks J, Klein L, Te AE. Title Pseudodyssynergia (contraction of the external sphincter during voiding) misdiagnosed as chronic nonbacterial prostatitis and the role of biofeedback as a therapeutic option. J Urol. 1997;157(6):2234–7.

Leskinen M, Lukkarinen O, Mattila T. Effects of finasteride in patients with inflammatory chronic pelvic pain syndrome: a double blind, placebo controlled, pilot study. Urology. 1999;53: 502–5.

Nickel JC, Downey J, Feliciano AEJ, Hennenfent B. Repetitive prostatic massage therapy for chronic refractory prostatitis: the Philippines experience. Tech Urol. 1999;5:146–51.

Nickel JC, Johnston B, Downey J, Barkin J, Pommerville P, Gregoire M, Ramsey E. Pentosan polysulfate therapy for chronic nonbacterial prostatitis (chronic pelvic pain syndrome category IIIA): a prospective multicenter clinical trial. Urology. 2000;56(3):413–7.

Paskiewicz E, Siegel S, Kirkemo A, Kirkpatrick C. Sacral nerve stimulation in patients with chronic intractable pelvic pain. J Urol. 2000;163(suppl):225 (abstract).

Wedren H. Effects of sodium pentosan polysulfate on symptoms related to chronic nonbacterial prostatitis. Scand J Urol Nephrol. 1987;21:81–8.

Chapter 30
STIs, Depression and Sexual Dysfunction

Calvin Fones

There is a relationship between STIs and sexual and mental health which is not immediately apparent to the practitioner. It may not have been there originally but develops subsequently in either the patient or his partner. The background of the patient is equally vital whether he/she is likely to develop problems. The inward-looking person is prone to develop depression if the "worry" of having had STI gets to him/her and people with strong religious upbringing carries the burden of "sinful deed" done, and if the partner gets terribly upset the patient may go into remorse that has led to suicides if he/she cannot come to terms with himself/herself. Three factors are important:

1. Behavioral risk factors and HIV/STI
2. Psychiatric morbidity and HIV/STI
3. Sexual disorders and HIV/STI

Behavioral Risk Factors and HIV/STI

- Sexual contact with multiple partners
- Low adherence to condom use
- Injected drug use or contact with injected drug users
- Unprotected sex between men
- Alcohol and drug abuse
- Depressive symptoms
- Recreational use of PDE5 agents

C. Fones, MBBS, M.D., FRCPsych, FAMS
National University of Singapore, Gleneagles Medical Centre, Gleneagles Hospital, Singapore, Singapore

Department of Psychiatry, National University Hospital, Singapore, Singapore
e-mail: pcmfslc@nus.edu.sg; fones@psychiatrist.sg

P.H.C. Lim (ed.), *Men's Health*,
DOI 10.1007/978-1-4471-4766-4_30, © Springer-Verlag London 2013

Psychiatric Morbidity and HIV/STI

- Psychological burden of HIV/STI
- Neuropsychiatric complications
- May affect adherence to treatments prescribed

Psychological Burden of HIV/STI

- Trauma of initial diagnosis
- Difficulty living with illness
- Ongoing threat of decline and effect on life expectancy
- Uncomfortable symptoms
- Lifestyle changes that are needed as a consequence of getting the disease
- Disability, if any, which is long term, e.g., urethral strictures and infertility
- Complicated therapeutic regimens sometimes needed, e.g., in AIDS patients
- Stigma
  - Guilt and poor self-esteem
  - Poor social support and isolation
  - Relationship difficulties

Neuropsychiatric Complications

- Neurosyphilis
- HIV encephalopathy
- CNS opportunistic infections
- Depression
- Mania
- Cognitive deficits and dementia

Adherence and Efficacy of Treatments

- Highly active antiretroviral therapy (HAART) may have neuropsychiatric effects:
  - Depression
  - Nervousness
  - Euphoria
  - Hallucinations/psychosis
- Help-seeking behavior may be reduced.
- Adherence to treatments may be compromised and reduced.

- Risk-reducing behaviors may be altered.
- Depression may impair cell-mediated immunity.

STI and Sexual Disorders

Patients often encounter temporary or more severe degrees of sexual dysfunction once they develop an STI, even if this has been cured. In those that leave a "permanent scar," e.g., herpes simplex, it often leads to protracted psychological problems which may include sexual dysfunction and even depression:

- History of STI affects sexual satisfaction later in life.
- History of STI quadruples a woman's chances of having painful intercourse and triples lubrication problems.
- Men are five times more likely to have unsatisfying sex life if they had an STD in the past.

History of STI and Sexual Anxiety

Having had STI the patient almost always develop some degree of anxiety leading to:

- Fear of reinfection
- Fear of infecting partner
- Performance anxiety during sex often develops:
  - Guilt
  - Anger and hostility
  - Avoidance

  There is significant emotional impact on the partner who may feel:

- Guilt and shame
- Blame
- Anger and betrayal
- Distress and depression
- Distrust
- Long remember the "betrayal"
- Adverse impact on the relationship/marriage

Treatment Options

- Treat underlying depression/anxiety.
- PDE5 inhibitor, e.g., Viagra, Cialis, or Levitra can be helpful for psychogenic ED.

- Psychotherapy may need several sessions.
- Individual therapy can be useful.
- Couple/marital relationship must be taken into consideration.
- Sex therapy—useful adjunct.

In concluding, this chapter is a reminder to the practitioner to be on the lookout for depression, sexual dysfunction, and other psychological disorders when they treat STIs.

Bibliography

Catalan J, Bradley M, Gallwey J, Hawton K. Sexual dysfunction and psychiatric morbidity in patients attending a clinic for sexually transmitted diseases. Br J Psychiatry. 1981;138:292–6.

Chen Y, et al. Depression associated with sexually transmitted infection in Canada. Sex Transm Infect. 2008;84:535–40.

Erbelding EJ, Hummel B, Hogan T, Zenilman J. High rates of depressive symptoms in STD clinic patients. J Sex Transm Dis. 2001;28(5):281–4.

Hutton HE, Lyketsos CG, Zenilman JM, Thompson RE, Erbelding EJ. Depression and HIV risk behaviors among patients in a sexually transmitted disease clinic. Am J Psychiatry. 2004;161(5): 912–4.

Jena AB. Sexually transmitted diseases among users of erectile dysfunction drugs: analysis of claims data. Ann Intern Med. 2010;153:1–7.

Sadeghi-Nejad H, Wasserman M, Weidner W, Richardson D, Goldmeier D. Sexually transmitted diseases and sexual function. J Sex Med. 2010;7(1 Pt 2):389–413.

Chapter 31
Guidelines: Making the Diagnosis and Managing the Partner

Peter Huat Chye Lim

Gonorrhea

(a) Purulent genital discharge (associated with dysuria in males) and history of recent unprotected sexual intercourse
(b) Gram-stained smear showing Gram-negative intracellular diplococci
(c) Culture positive for *N. gonorrhoeae*
(d) Nucleic acid amplification test (NAAT) (e.g., PCR) positive for *N. gonorrhoeae*

Nongonococcal Urethritis (NGU)

(a) Mucopurulent or whitish discharge from urethra associated with dysuria or urethral discomfort/itch in males and history of recent unprotected sexual intercourse
(b) Gram-stained smear showing increased pus cell count (five or more WBC per high-power field) in absence of Gram-negative intracellular diplococci
(c) Visible threads in the first glass of a 2-glass urine test

P.H.C. Lim, MBBS, MMed(Surg), M.Inst.Urol(Lon) FAMS, D.Urol(Lon), FICS
Andrology Urology & Continence Centre, Gleneagles Hospital, Singapore, Singapore

H.T. Naval Medical School, Surabaya, Indonesia

Edith Cowan University, Joondalup, WA, Australia

Society for Men's Health Singapore, Midview City, Singapore

Gleneagles Medical Centre, Singapore, Singapore

Department of Urology, Changi General Hospital, Singapore, Singapore
e-mail: profpeter.lim@gmail.com

P.H.C. Lim (ed.), *Men's Health*,
DOI 10.1007/978-1-4471-4766-4_31,

Chlamydia Genital Infection

(a) Nucleic acid amplification test (NAAT) (e.g., PCR) positive for *C. trachomatis* from anogenital specimen
(b) Antigen detection (e.g., EIA, IF) positive for *C. trachomatis* from anogenital specimen

Infectious Syphilis

(a) Presence of primary chancre usually solitary, indurated, non-tender (but the ulcer may also be atypical) and inguinal lymphadenopathy
(b) Presence of clinical features of secondary syphilis, e.g., rash especially on palms and soles, anogenital patches and growths, generalized lymphadenopathy, and patchy hair loss

Confirmed by:
Positive dark-ground microscopic examination for spirochaetes
Reactive blood tests for syphilis:

(i) Screening test (RPR/VDRL)
(ii) Confirmatory tests (TPPA/TPHA, LIA, EIA)

Noninfectious Syphilis

(a) Presence of clinical features of tertiary syphilis (viz., cardiovascular syphilis and central nervous system syphilis)
(b) Asymptomatic infection with reactive blood tests for syphilis
    (i) Screening test (RPR/VDRL)
    (ii) Confirmatory tests (TPPA/TPHA, LIA, EIA)

Note: Persistence of reactive serology in patients with treated syphilis may be indicative of a serological scar.

Congenital Syphilis

(a) Presence of clinical features of active disease (e.g., mucocutaneous signs, hepatosplenomegaly, bone changes)
    Confirmed by reactive blood tests for syphilis:
    (i) Screening test (RPR/VDRL)
    (ii) Confirmatory tests (TPPA/TPHA, LIA, EIA)

(b) Asymptomatic infection in infant born to infected mother with:

   (i) Detectable LIA IgM in infant.
   (ii) RPR/VDRL titer in infant fourfold or greater than in mother.
   (iii) RPR/VDRL titer shows serial rise.
   (iv) Reactive CSF-VDRL or abnormal CSF FEME in infant.

Genital Herpes (First Episode)

(a) Typical lesions (usually severe) of genital herpes appearing for the first time on the genitals

Confirmed by viral isolation, PCR, EIA, or type-specific serological test for HSV that indicates seroconversion.

Provide information on type of HSV detected where available.

Genital Herpes (Recurrent)

(a) Typical lesions of genital herpes occurring in a patient with a history of previous attacks of genital herpes

Confirmed by viral isolation, PCR, EIA, or type-specific serological test for HSV.

Provide information on type of HSV detected where available.

Repeat notifications of recurrent genital herpes are not necessary.

Managing the Partner

Should be appropriate for the identified or suspected STD. Partners should be notified, examined, and treated for the STD identified or suspected in the index patient.

Partners should be instructed to abstain from sexual intercourse until they and their sex partners are cured. In the absence of a microbiological test of cure, this means when therapy has been completed and patient and partner(s) are asymptomatic.

Bibliography

Guidelines for Treatment of Sexually Transmitted Diseases; CDC MMWR Recommendations & Reports; Vol. 47/No. RR-1. 9–122.

Fluoroquinolones No Longer Recommended for Treatment of Gonococcal Infections. http://www.cdc.gov/mmwr/preview/mmwrhtml/mm5614a3.htm. Accessed on 6 Dec 2012.

French P. UK National Guidelines on the Management of late syphilis & other STI's. 2002. http://www.Bashh.org/guidelines/.

Ministry of Health, Singapore: Recommendations to Registered Medical Practitioners. Chapter 137 Reg 2 MD131 Section 6 (1) IDA MOH Directive 3A/2008. Notification of Sexually Transmitted Infections (Guidelines in Diagnosis) Annexe B.

Adler M, Cowan F, French P, editors. ABC of sexually transmitted infections. 5th ed. BMJ Publ. Group; 2004. ISBN 0-7279-17517.

Index

P.H.C. Lim (ed.), *Men's Health*,
DOI 10.1007/978-1-4471-4766-4, © Springer-Verlag London 2013

Printed by Publishers' Graphics LLC
AMZ20130210.19.19.78